Prediabetes Diet and Action Plan

PREDIABETES

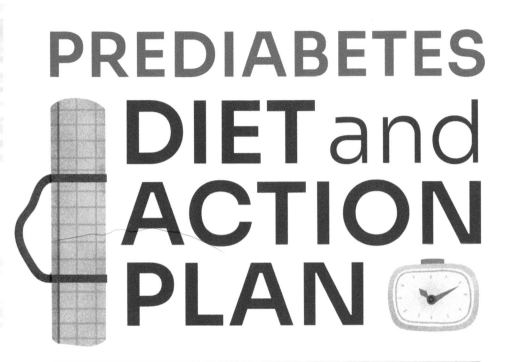

DIET and ACTION PLAN

A Guide to Reverse Prediabetes and Start New Healthy Habits

ALICE FIGUEROA, MPH, RDN, CDN

ROCKRIDGE
PRESS

For general information on our other products and services or to obtain technical support, please contact our Customer Care Department within the United States at (866) 744-2665, or outside the United States at (510) 253-0500.

Rockridge Press publishes its books in a variety of electronic and print formats. Some content that appears in print may not be available in electronic books, and vice versa.

Interior and Cover Designer: Jane Archer
Art Producer: Sara Feinstein
Editor: Rebecca Markley
Production Editor: Emily Sheehan
Production Manager: Jose Olivera

Illustration © 2021 Clare Owen, cover, p. iii, vi, 2, 16, 21, 32, 42, 56, 72, 86, 108, 130; © 2020 James Pop, pp, 36-39. Author photo courtesy of Patrick Kolts.

ISBN: Print 978-1-64876-519-3 | eBook 978-1-64876-520-9
R1

To my brother **Isaac**, who inspires me to cook and care for my patients with kindness and joy; to my parents, **Enrique and Maria Teresa**, who migrated to the United States and worked tirelessly to nurture my passion for public health; and to my brother **Enrique**, who left this life too soon but who remains an eternal source of inspiration.

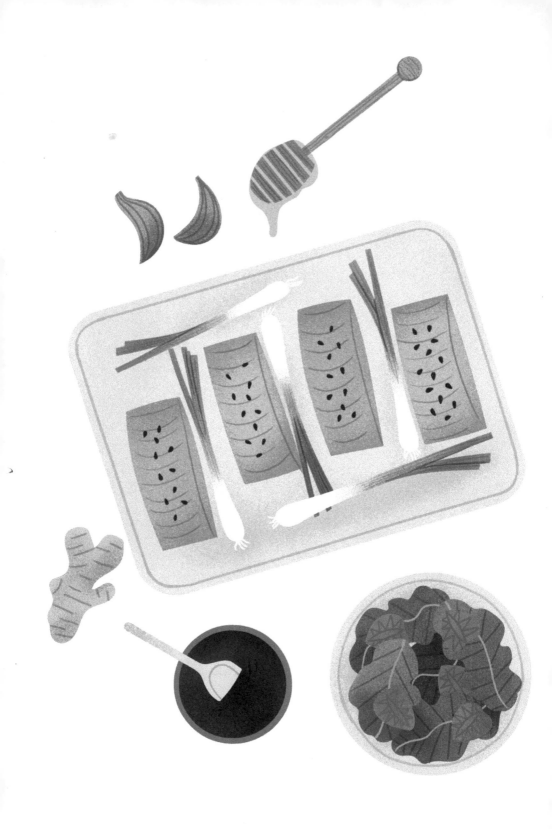

Contents

Introduction

Reversal of prediabetes is within your reach at any size, body shape, or health status. If you've been diagnosed with prediabetes, you may be feeling concerned and lost as to how to control your blood sugar and reclaim your health. Perhaps you've been told by your doctor and health team that you need to improve your lifestyle and change your diet to prevent the onset of diabetes. You may be asking yourself, "How do I change my lifestyle and diet?" As a registered dietitian, nutritionist, public health researcher, and diabetes prevention lifestyle coach, I've developed a prediabetes reversal guide that will allow you to sustainably reverse prediabetes, improve your quality of life, and maximize your health. I have spent more than a decade working with patients and clients who've been diagnosed with metabolic, endocrine, and cardiovascular conditions including prediabetes, diabetes, heart disease, hypertension, and high cholesterol. The patients and clients who used my prediabetes reversal guide have successfully lowered their HgA1C, blood sugar levels, cholesterol, and blood pressure. In addition to seeing improvements in their metabolic and cardiac health, the patients and clients I've supported have been able to stop using restrictive diets and disordered eating behaviors that are unsustainable, unrealistic, and harmful to their mental and physical health. Instead, they've felt empowered to embrace a liberating lifestyle and nutrition philosophy that promotes health and happiness. My prediabetes reversal guide has three pillars:

Pillar 1: Nourishment through Mindful & Intuitive Eating and Plant-Based Nutrition
Pillar 2: Movement
Pillar 3: Stress Reduction through Mindfulness

I was also inspired to design delicious and health-supportive recipes after my parents were diagnosed with prediabetes and other metabolic conditions that required them to make changes to their diets. After learning about their prediabetes diagnosis, my parents immediately thought that they would need to give up their favorite foods. My parents are not alone in their fear. When patients initially seek my support, they are also fearful that the only way to manage prediabetes is to eat bland and boring diet food. My mission is to create scrumptious, culturally rich food that supports your health, helps you reverse prediabetes, and satisfies your cravings for delicious food. My mother successfully reversed prediabetes and my dad improved his A1C levels after adopting the mindful, plant-based eating philosophy presented in this book. They didn't have to give up delicious food, and neither will you.

You'll find that the recipes in this book are influenced by Latin American culinary traditions and Creole cuisine. Inspired by my Guatemalan heritage and New Orleans upbringing, my cooking style champions fresh produce, aromatic herbs and spices, and comfort food. I've also been blessed to spend time in Italy, South Africa, Costa Rica, Thailand, and India learning about nutrition, public health, Ayurveda, yoga, and food studies. I treasure and honor the diverse food traditions I've learned about by infusing them into my cooking. I hope that you'll also enjoy learning about diverse ingredients and exploring new cooking techniques and food flavors in your kitchen.

In this book, you will learn how to implement realistic and easy-to-incorporate changes in your lifestyle that will motivate you to move your body and calm your mind. You will also be provided with all the tools needed to reverse prediabetes through mindful eating and plant-based nutrition including a meal plan, recipes, and nutritional recommendations. With this book, my goal is to support you every step of the way as you rediscover the power you have to take charge of your well-being. Think of this book as your guide to empowering yourself to reverse prediabetes and reclaim your health.

part I

Foundations of Prediabetes Reversal

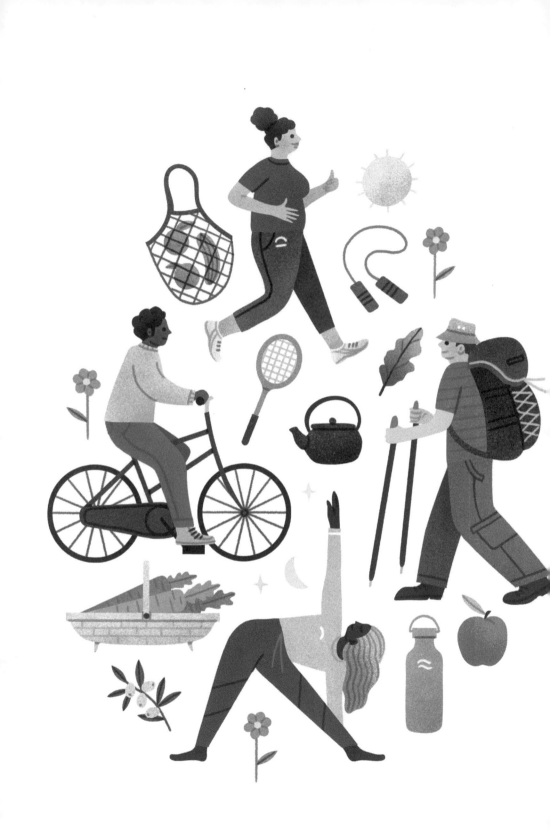

CHAPTER 1

What You Need to Know about Prediabetes

Prediabetes is a metabolic condition affecting children and adults of all ages that occurs when blood sugar (glucose) levels, also known as glycemic levels, are higher than normal but not yet elevated enough to be diagnosed as diabetes. A review of multiple studies on prediabetes published in the journal *Clinical Diabetes and Endocrinology* confirmed that without implementing lifestyle and nutrition changes, 10 to 25 percent of individuals with prediabetes will develop type 2 diabetes within three to five years and 70 percent of people diagnosed with prediabetes will progress to have type 2 diabetes (also known as diabetes mellitus) within their lifetime. Since prediabetes is most often symptom-free, it may progress for years without being diagnosed. Globally, 352.1 million individuals between the ages of 20 and 79 have prediabetes, which accounts for 7.3 percent of the world's adult population. In the United States, more than one in three adults, or about 88 million people, have prediabetes.

Prediabetes may have few to no symptoms, but it puts you at a higher risk of developing serious health complications including stroke, heart disease, and type 2 diabetes. According to the National Institutes of Health (NIH) MedlinePlus website, complications due to type 2 diabetes include damaged blood vessels and nerves in the cardiovascular, digestive, genital, urinary, motor, and metabolic systems. If prediabetes is allowed to turn into diabetes, you will also be at a higher risk for heart, kidney, eye, skin, foot, and gum diseases. Although prediabetes is a condition that requires care and attention, it is crucial for you to keep a positive outlook and understand that you have the power to reverse prediabetes by making realistic, attainable changes to your lifestyle and diet. You can stop the progression of prediabetes and prevent diabetes and the health complications that result from it.

Take your prediabetes diagnosis as an opportunity to be kind to yourself, take charge of your health, and be proactive in preventing diabetes. The more you understand about how the body manages blood sugar, the more empowered you will be to reverse prediabetes. Let's break down the science behind blood sugar and prediabetes.

Understanding Insulin Resistance

Prediabetes develops when the body is unable to properly use a hormone called insulin to metabolize, absorb, and balance blood sugar. Insulin is produced by the pancreas, and its production is connected to the amount of carbohydrates, protein, and fat we eat. When we eat food that contains carbohydrates, the digestive system breaks down carbohydrates into glucose, which is a type of naturally occurring sugar. Glucose is a simple sugar that is absorbed into the bloodstream through the lining of the small intestine. When the body's glucose levels rise, insulin is released from the pancreas into the bloodstream. The main role of insulin is to absorb glucose from the bloodstream and either use it for energy or store it in the liver and muscles for later use.

Insulin resistance is one of the main contributing factors to the development of prediabetes and diabetes. Insulin resistance occurs when the fat, muscle, and liver cells no longer respond efficiently to insulin. As a result, the body is unable to absorb glucose from the bloodstream. To compensate, the pancreas then begins to make excess insulin. Prediabetes occurs when the pancreas cannot produce sufficient insulin to maintain balanced blood glucose levels within a normal range and/or when the cells in the body become resistant to insulin. If the body is unable to keep up with insulin demand, glucose will remain in the blood, causing elevated blood sugar levels and the development of type 2 diabetes over time.

You may find it surprising to learn that insulin resistance and high blood sugar may also affect your metabolic and heart health. In addition to managing carbohydrate metabolism, insulin also regulates how fat and protein are used and stored in the body. As a result, individuals with insulin resistance may be at a higher risk of developing metabolic syndrome. Metabolic syndrome is a group of conditions that place you at risk for cardiovascular and metabolic conditions such as prediabetes, type 2 diabetes, heart disease, and stroke. The conditions associated with metabolic syndrome are high blood pressure, high blood sugar, excess fat around the abdominal area, and elevated triglyceride and cholesterol levels. To better understand why there is a connection between insulin resistance and overall metabolic and cardiac health, we must first learn that insulin plays a role in fat absorption and storage. Prediabetes and insulin resistance are associated with high cholesterol and triglyceride levels. Insulin also affects how the protein we eat is absorbed, stored, and broken down. In later chapters, we will learn the roles that protein and fat play in helping you maintain healthy blood sugar levels.

Reversing Insulin Resistance

The good news is that lifestyle and dietary choices can improve prediabetes and reduce insulin resistance. Lifestyle changes that you can make to reverse insulin resistance include:

Adopting a mindful movement practice. Physical activity leads to improved glycemic (blood sugar) control, reduced insulin resistance, and improved use of insulin that allows for more efficient absorption of sugar in the bloodstream. Regular physical activity is also linked to a decrease in inflammatory fat and greater cardiovascular fitness, which both contribute to improved insulin function.

Increasing your consumption of fiber-rich vegetables and fruits. Foods with a low glycemic index may help prevent the progression of insulin resistance. A systematic meta-analysis of diabetes research published in the journal *PLoS Medicine* concluded that a high-fiber diet results in reduced levels of cholesterol, LDL cholesterol (bad cholesterol), and triglycerides. Lowering high levels of lipids improves management of insulin resistance and hyperglycemia (high blood sugar levels). Adding more fiber to your diet also helps improve HbA1c and fasting glucose levels, which are labs used to diagnose prediabetes. A good goal is to increase fiber intake by about 15 grams per day until you reach at least 35 to 45 grams of daily fiber intake.

Practicing stress reduction techniques like meditation, deep breathing, and mindfulness. Stress can lead to the release of cortisol and other stress hormones that cause an increase in blood glucose levels. Furthermore, a reduction of stress can help you find the time, space, and motivation to make dietary, physical activity, and self-care decisions that nurture your overall well-being.

Choosing whole foods and non-sugary drinks. Foods that are highly processed tend to be high in sugar, saturated fats, and artificial sweeteners, which all contribute to insulin resistance and prediabetes.

Making time for rest and sleep. Aim to sleep for seven hours or more each night. Poor or insufficient sleep is associated with higher blood sugar levels, which leads to insulin resistance over time. Include rest and downtime in your daily schedule.

Risk Factors and Diagnosis

Risk factors for prediabetes and insulin resistance can be classified into three categories: hereditary, acquired, and a mixture of both hereditary and acquired causes. Hereditary causes are biological traits that are passed from one generation to another within a family. Examples of hereditary causes include genetic medical conditions such as lipodystrophy (irregular distribution of fat within the body), polycystic ovarian syndrome (PCOS), and type A and type B insulin resistance.

Acquired causes are typically related to lifestyle and include imbalanced nutrition, physical inactivity, smoking, not getting enough sleep, and taking certain medications such as glucocorticoids, antipsychotics, antiadrenergic agents, protease inhibitors, and exogenous insulin.

Sugar and the Glycemic Index

When we eat and digest food, our blood sugar increases. Foods rich in carbohydrates including fruit, grains, legumes, dairy, and vegetables all affect our blood sugar levels. Why do carbohydrates affect blood sugar levels? Let's say you eat an apple. When you bite into an apple and chew it, the saliva in your mouth begins the process of digestion as it breaks down the apple. The chewed apple then travels down your esophagus and into your stomach and small intestine, where it is fully digested. Once the apple is digested, it is broken down into sugars. The sugars produced from digested carbohydrates are released into the bloodstream.

The glycemic index rates food on a scale from 1 to 100 based on how slowly or quickly a food raises blood sugar. Foods ranked high on the glycemic index scale are quickly digested and absorbed, causing a rapid release of sugar into the bloodstream. High glycemic index foods and drinks include simple carbohydrates like sodas, sports drinks, pastries, and all foods high in added sugar. The body digests low glycemic foods more efficiently and at a slower rate. Low glycemic foods release sugar slowly into the bloodstream and lead to a steady rise of blood sugar and balanced blood sugar levels. Low glycemic index foods include complex carbohydrates like pumpernickel bread, beans, lentils, leafy vegetables, squashes, berries, and apples. A diet rich in low glycemic index foods supports healthy blood sugar levels and helps reverse prediabetes and insulin resistance.

Many people who are diagnosed with prediabetes have a combination of hereditary and acquired risk factors. If any of these risk factors apply to you, it is important to be screened regularly for prediabetes.

FACTORS BEYOND YOUR CONTROL

Many of the contributing factors for prediabetes are not modifiable through lifestyle changes. It is important to find well-being practices to reduce distress, depression, or anxiety that may arise after learning about prediabetes factors that are beyond your control. A study published in the *Journal of Diabetes Research* examined the effects of positive psychology on managing diabetes and prediabetes and found that finding ways to increase your optimism, well-being, and resiliency and develop positive emotions is crucial to gently and effectively managing prediabetes and achieving better health.

Age

As you get older, the risk of developing prediabetes increases. According to the Centers for Disease Control and Prevention (CDC), about one in three adults in the United States has prediabetes, and most of those adults are over the age of 45. While the number of young adults, adolescents, and children diagnosed with prediabetes is unfortunately increasing, older adults are more likely to develop diabetes. This is largely due to increased insulin resistance and decreased pancreatic efficiency caused by loss of muscle mass (sarcopenia), high fat body composition (adiposity), and low physical activity levels.

Genetics

Hereditary factors passed on within families can increase the risk of prediabetes. Having a first-degree blood relative (parent or sibling) with diabetes may increase prediabetes risk. Other genetic medical conditions such as lipodystrophy, PCOS, and Type A and Type B insulin resistance are also risk factors for prediabetes. Less common genetic risk factors include Werner syndrome, Rabson-Mendenhall syndrome, Alström syndrome, ataxia-telangiectasia, and myotonic dystrophy. Mapping out your family's health history can help you determine if you are at an increased risk. Make sure to share your family's diabetes history with your doctors so they can develop a prediabetes screening process tailored to your specific needs. According to the American Diabetes Association, prediabetes often runs in families due to genetic traits, shared environmental factors, common lifestyle choices, and similar eating and exercise habits. You can use the chart on page 10 to document your family's health history.

Gestational Diabetes

Being diagnosed with gestational diabetes or giving birth to a baby who weighs nine pounds or more can place you at an increased risk of developing prediabetes. Gestational diabetes occurs during pregnancy in women who do not have diabetes prior to being pregnant. During pregnancy, natural changes in weight and hormones cause the body to use insulin less effectively, sometimes resulting in the development of insulin resistance. Individuals with gestational diabetes do not produce sufficient insulin to promote healthy blood glucose levels. Babies who are exposed to high blood glucose levels and maternal insulin resistance in utero may suffer from added stress to the pancreas, leading to an increased risk of prediabetes and insulin abnormalities later in life. Gestational diabetes is an early symptom of irregular insulin function and can progress to type 2 diabetes. You can learn more about gestational diabetes at CDC.gov/diabetes/basics/gestational.html.

Race or Ethnic Background

Although prevalence of prediabetes is similar across all ethnic and social groups, Black, Indigenous, and People of Color (BIPOC) have a greater chance of developing diabetes due to genetic predispositions, health disparities, and various environmental factors. Members of BIPOC communities may experience barriers that make it more difficult to prevent and manage diabetes, such as lack of access to culturally sensitive health care that empowers individuals to make positive behavioral changes.

Medical Conditions

Being diagnosed with certain medical conditions can put you at a higher risk of developing prediabetes. The following medical conditions are associated with increased risk of developing prediabetes: high blood pressure (hypertension), high cholesterol, gestational diabetes, metabolic syndrome, heart disease or stroke, and PCOS. If you manage

my **family health** portrait

Name: _____ **Date:** _____

Grandmother	Grandfather

_____
_____
_____

_____
_____
_____

Aunts/Uncles   Mother

_____   _____   _____   _____
_____   _____   _____   _____
_____   _____   _____   _____

Brothers/Sisters   **You**

_____   _____   _____
_____   _____   _____
_____   _____   _____

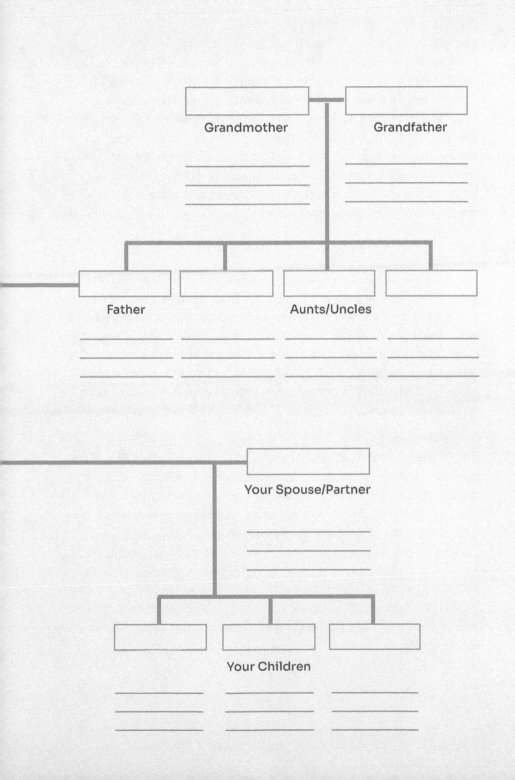

Grandmother

Grandfather

Father

Aunts/Uncles

Your Spouse/Partner

Your Children

any of these chronic conditions, it is important to be screened regularly for prediabetes.

Assigned or Biological Sex

Being assigned as male at birth places you at a higher risk of prediabetes. According to CDC statistics, 37.4 percent of men have prediabetes versus 29.2 percent of women living in the United States. Several large studies have indicated that men tend to develop prediabetes at lower weights when compared to women and are more likely to store adipose tissue (fat around the organs). These same studies suggest that men may also be less sensitive to insulin, meaning that they are not able to use insulin as well to absorb blood sugar efficiently. While these theories are still being researched, we do know that men are more likely than women to be diagnosed with prediabetes.

FACTORS WITHIN YOUR CONTROL

You have the ability to reverse prediabetes. Although there are many factors that cannot be altered, we know that lifestyle changes can make a big difference. The purpose of this book is to provide you with the knowledge, practices, meal plan, and recipes needed to empower you to adopt lasting lifestyle changes that will improve your overall health. In order to succeed, it is essential for you to believe in your ability to make positive changes and adopt behaviors that consider your food preferences as well as your cultural and wellness needs.

What You Eat

The food you eat directly affects your blood glucose levels. Therefore, it is important to increase your consumption of foods that support balanced glycemic control and manage your intake of foods that make it more difficult to maintain healthy blood glucose levels. Eating excess amounts of simple sugars and high glycemic index foods will cause sharp spikes in blood sugar. Spikes in blood sugar can lead to abnormal blood sugar stability (dysglycemia). When blood sugar levels are unstable, you may experience hyperglycemia (high blood sugar) and hypoglycemia (low blood sugar). Over time, these sharp fluctuations can damage the systems used to secrete insulin and absorb blood sugar.

How Much You Move Your Body

Physical inactivity is one of the leading contributors to the development of prediabetes and diabetes, and the World Health Organization estimates that up to 5 million global deaths annually could be prevented if people were more active. Physical activity aids in the management of insulin resistance by helping your body become more sensitive to insulin. This helps your tissues absorb blood glucose more efficiently. Moving your body also helps balance blood sugar and reduces the risk of heart disease and other metabolic conditions that negatively impact your blood sugar and overall health.

How Much You Sleep

Poor sleep quality, insufficient sleep, and sleep disorders like sleep apnea and insomnia are linked to increased risk of prediabetes. Studies have found that sleep deprivation can lead to insulin resistance and glucose intolerance (a term used to describe conditions like prediabetes that result in high blood glucose). A research article published in *Diabetes Care* linked short sleep duration to metabolic imbalances, heart disease, irregular appetite, and overactive immune and inflammatory responses. Not getting a good night's sleep may also lead to poor eating habits, like unnecessary nighttime snacking or increased alcohol consumption.

Smoking

The more cigarettes you smoke, the higher risk you have of developing prediabetes and type 2 diabetes. Smokers have a 30 to 40 percent higher chance of developing diabetes than nonsmokers. Smoking is associated with increased adipose (fat tissue) around the abdominal area and organs. Studies conducted by the *International Journal of Clinical Practice* and the Cardiovascular and Metabolic Diseases Etiology Research Center concluded that having excess fat around the organs increases the release of inflammatory proteins that are linked to increased risk of developing insulin resistance, hypertension (high blood pressure), arterial disease, and high triglycerides and cholesterol levels. Smoking also leads to oxidative stress, a condition that occurs when harmful chemicals in cigarettes cause cellular damage. If you are currently a smoker, it is never too late to quit. Quitting at any age is beneficial to your health. Studies show that after just eight weeks of quitting cigarettes, your body uses insulin more efficiently, leading to improved blood sugar levels. Here are some tips to help you along:

- List the reasons why you want to quit smoking. What is your motivation?
- Think about the benefits of quitting: saving money, better lung function, reduced risk of prediabetes, and so on.
- Set a date to quit smoking. Try to give yourself at least a two-week window so you can adjust to the idea and set expectations. Pick a time that is not too stressful for you.
- Throw out all cigarettes, e-cigarettes, and tobacco products.
- Connect to your social support system including family, friends, and colleagues when you are ready to quit. Find supportive loved ones to keep you accountable and motivated.
- Anticipate and plan for the challenges that will arise, including nicotine withdrawal and cravings.
- Find a way to cope with cravings, like exercising, deep breathing, meditation, walking, or talking to a loved one.
- Talk to your health team about quitting. Let your doctor, therapist, social worker, and dietitian know that you are quitting. They may be able to provide you with medications, smoking cessation therapy, relaxation techniques, and behavioral practices to help you quit.

DIAGNOSING PREDIABETES

Prediabetes has few to no symptoms, and as a result, the majority of people with prediabetes do not know that they have it. However, there are some subtle symptoms that have been linked to prediabetes. According to the American Academy of Dermatology Association, people with prediabetes may experience acanthosis nigricans, a condition that causes darkening of the skin around the neck and armpits, and they may also develop small skin tags, which are benign skin growths, around the eye, neck, groin, and armpit area. Skin tags develop due to excess blood sugar and insulin in the body.

Since symptoms for prediabetes are not easy to pinpoint, it is important to have good communication with your medical team so that they can assess your risk of developing prediabetes based on family history, medical history, and lifestyle. It is also crucial for you to be honest with yourself and become your own health advocate. If you know that you don't regularly engage in physical activity and/or your diet is low in fruits and vegetables and/or high in highly processed foods and simple sugars, it is beneficial to be screened regularly. The National Institute of Diabetes and Digestive and Kidney Diseases recommends three types of screening tests: A1C, fasting plasma glucose, and a two-hour post 75 g oral glucose challenge.

The A1C and fasting plasma tests are conducted through a simple blood test. For the fasting plasma test, you will need to not eat or drink anything except water for eight hours before the test, so it is recommended that you conduct this test early in the morning. A1C assesses long-term management of blood glucose and doesn't require fasting, since it measures average blood levels for the previous two to three months. The two-hour oral glucose challenge measures blood sugar after drinking a sweet drink. It allows doctors to evaluate how well your body is processing glucose. Elevated results in one or more of these tests can be used to diagnose prediabetes.

Making Changes

I want to take this opportunity to remind you that no matter what shape you're in right now, you can make lifestyle and nutrition changes that can help you manage insulin resistance, reverse prediabetes, and reclaim your health. In this book, we will embark on a wellness journey together that will provide you with the tools needed to achieve your goals in a way that seamlessly fits into your everyday life. This book is not another fad diet that will ask you to restrict eating so much that you're left feeling hungry, dissatisfied, or bad about yourself. Together we will explore how to make sustainable, affordable, realistic, and practical lifestyle changes that will help you succeed in managing or reversing prediabetes. The meal plan and recipes in this book are designed to nourish your body and satisfy your craving for delicious, zesty food.

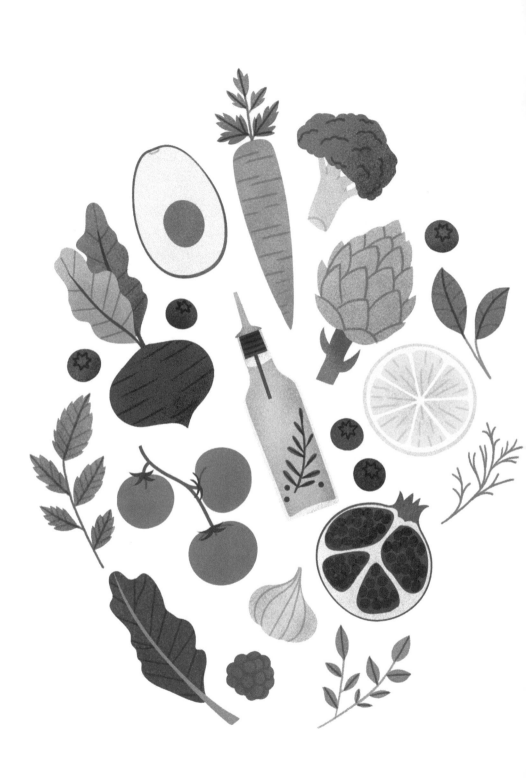

CHAPTER 2

Nutrition and Prediabetes

At this point, you may be thinking that making healthy changes to your diet is too difficult or even unattainable. However, I come bearing wonderful news! Eating healthy does not need to be complicated, restrictive, or boring, and you don't need to feel intimidated about having the perfect diet. Being healthy is about practice, not perfection. In this chapter, you will learn how to use food to reverse prediabetes and bring healing to your body. You will explore the proven benefits of adopting a plant-based diet and mindful eating practices. You will learn how to implement realistic and practical nutrition changes into your daily schedule. This chapter serves as the ultimate nutrition guide to reversing prediabetes.

How Healthy Nutrition Helps Reversal

The food we eat affects our blood sugar levels and risk of developing prediabetes. The body needs a balanced intake of micronutrients and macronutrients to produce energy, repair cells, and maintain health. Micronutrients include vitamins and minerals, whereas macronutrients include carbohydrates, fats, and proteins. Carbohydrates provide energy for the central nervous system (including the brain), fuel our muscles, and support other bodily functions. In addition, carbohydrates provide fiber, an indigestible substance found in fruits and vegetables that promotes healthy digestion, keeps you full and satisfied after eating, and helps maintain regular bowel movements and balanced blood sugar levels. Fats provide fuel for energy, aid in the absorption and production of vitamins and hormones, and regulate body temperature. Proteins are needed for the growth, maintenance, and repair of the body and are crucial to hormone and immune health. These three macronutrients work together to provide the necessary nourishment and calories for optimal bodily functioning. A healthy diet needs all three of these macronutrients.

CARBS ARE NOT THE ENEMY

It may be surprising for you to learn that carbohydrates are naturally occurring sugar molecules that are linked together. Natural sugars, when eaten as a part of a well-balanced diet, are not unhealthy. In fact, the natural sugars that make up carbohydrates provide support for maintaining the health of our cell structures and fuel for optimal brain and body function. Although many popular fad diets villainize carbohydrates as the culprits for diabetes and other diet-related chronic conditions, carbohydrates are actually good for you!

There are two categories of carbohydrates: complex and simple carbohydrates. Myths about carbohydrates fail to recognize that some of the most health-supportive foods are complex carbohydrates, including all fruits, vegetables, and whole grains. Complex carbohydrates are rich in fiber and, as a result, are more slowly digested and absorbed by the body. This leads to more efficient insulin function and balanced blood sugar levels. Simple carbohydrates do not have much fiber, which causes them to be rapidly digested and absorbed by the body. Excess intake of simple carbohydrates can lead to insulin resistance, sugar spikes, unbalanced blood sugar levels, and hyperglycemia (high blood sugar). All added sugars (sugars that are added to foods and drinks when they are prepared, cooked, or processed) are simple sugars. Examples of added sugars include refined white sugar, corn syrup, brown sugar, honey, maple syrup, molasses, and agave nectar. Excess intake of foods and drinks rich in added sugars can lead to insulin resistance and prediabetes.

Focus on Healthy Carbs

The best sources for healthy, fiber-rich carbohydrates are vegetables, fruits, whole grains, and legumes. These foods are excellent sources of antioxidants, vitamins, minerals, and fiber needed to support overall health. Practicing a plant-based diet, in which complex carbohydrates make up the majority of your diet, has been shown to be the most sustainable and efficient way to manage prediabetes. A good way to make sure you are practicing a plant-based diet is to make sure you eat non-starchy vegetables and fruits at most meals on a daily basis.

Fresh, frozen, and canned vegetables and fruits are all great options, and I encourage you to purchase vegetables and fruits that work for your food preferences and budget. When choosing grains, I recommend that you eat mostly whole grains. These include 100 percent whole-wheat pasta and bread, quinoa, farro, millet, bulgur, and rice. Although brown rice has a slightly lower glycemic index than white rice, if you prefer to eat white rice, go for it. (We will discuss the appropriate portion sizes for whole-grain carbohydrates a bit later.) Legumes such as beans, peanuts, lentils, and peas are also excellent sources of protein and healthy carbohydrates.

DAILY NUTRITIONAL GOALS

Here is a list of my mindful eating pillars, which provide guidelines to reverse prediabetes.

- Replace ultra-processed foods like hot dogs with fresh whole foods like roasted salmon or chickpea stew.
- Add healthy fats like avocados and seeds to your plate and limit intake of foods high in saturated and trans fats such as butter and shortening. Limit intake of deep-fried foods and replace with foods that are lightly sautéed in olive oil.
- Swap out refined grains like white sandwich bread for fiber-rich whole grains like pumpernickel bread or 100 percent whole-wheat bread. You may still enjoy mindful portions of refined grains, but our goal is to increase intake of whole grains.
- Limit intake of foods high in added sugars like white sugar and corn syrup and sugar substitutes like Splenda and Sweet'N Low. Foods high in added sugars and sugar substitutes include soft drinks, sports drinks, and desserts. Keep in mind that many added sugars are hidden in seemingly healthy foods like flavored yogurt, salad dressings, and canned soups.

- Choose foods with low amounts of added salt. Foods that are high in salt include fast food and frozen meals. Closely read the nutrition labels and compare the amount of sodium in foods such as soup, bread, and frozen meals. Choose foods with low amounts of sodium.
- A healthy diet consists of replacing low-nutrient, high-calorie foods with nutrient-rich, high-fiber foods for most of your meals and snacks. Make healthier snacking choices by swapping chips for hummus, vegetable sticks, and a small 100 percent whole-wheat pita bread. You may still eat chips occasionally, but our focus is to add more nutritious foods to your daily diet.

The Balanced Plate

A health-supportive diet includes a balanced intake of complex carbohydrates, healthy fats, and lean proteins. A simple way to make sure your plate is balanced at each meal is to follow the **My Plate: Prediabetes Reversal Method** based on the Centers for Disease Control and Prevention Prevent T2 program, which can be found at CDC .gov/diabetes/prevention/index.html. Additional nutritional information can be found at Diabetes.org/healthy-living/recipes-nutrition. The following guidelines are based on information from these two sources.

- Fill half of your plate with complex, non-starchy carbohydrates like green leafy vegetables, cruciferous vegetables, eggplant, carrots, celery, mushrooms, okra, zucchini, and Brussels sprouts.
- Fill a quarter of your plate with lean proteins like beans, tofu, tuna, eggs, chicken, or salmon.
- Fill a quarter of your plate with whole-grain carbohydrates like quinoa, rice, bulgur, oatmeal, or whole-wheat bread.
- To add nutrient-rich fat to your meal, I also recommend that you include a healthy fat component like avocado, nuts, seeds, olives, yogurt, or cheese. Healthy fat helps you feel satiated and full for longer. Adding healthy fats to your plate has been linked to reduced risk of developing type 2 diabetes and other cardiovascular diseases.
- Fruit is an excellent source of soluble and insoluble fiber, and as a result, it does not cause drastic spikes in blood sugar levels. To add

my plate: prediabetes reversal method

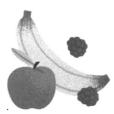

Portion of Fruit

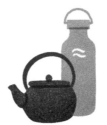

Water or Drink with no added sugar

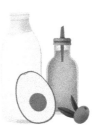

Portion of Fat

Grains and Starchy Veggies

Non-starchy Veggies

Protein Foods

more fiber and antioxidants to your meal, you may also include a small to medium serving of fruit such as a banana, ½ to 1 cup of berries, or an apple. You can eat more fruit at breakfast if you are not eating non-starchy veggies. It is recommended that people with prediabetes, diabetes, and the general population eat at least 1 to 2 cups of fruit per day.

- Make sure to drink water or beverages with no added sugars or artificial sweeteners like unsweetened hot or iced tea, unsweetened coffee, or seltzer water. I do not recommend regularly drinking diet drinks that contain artificial sweeteners. Although artificial sweeteners reduce calories, their consumption has not been linked to any long-term health benefits like improved blood glucose levels.

½ PLATE = NON-STARCHY VEGETABLES

Vegetables fall into two categories: starchy and non-starchy. Both starchy and non-starchy vegetables provide vitamins, minerals, fiber, and antioxidants and should be included in your diet. Starchy vegetables have a higher glycemic index, meaning that they cause your blood sugar to increase more after eating when compared to non-starchy vegetables. You can eat some starchy vegetables on a daily basis as a part of your healthy starch/whole-grain starch carbohydrate intake, but you'll want most of your vegetables to be non-starchy. Non-starchy vegetables have a very low glycemic index and are rich in fiber. As a result, you can eat larger portions of non-starchy vegetables to help you feel more satisfied and full without risking an increase in blood sugar levels. The goal is to eat at least three to five servings of non-starchy vegetables per day. The more vegetables you eat, the better for your health.

¼ PLATE = LEAN PROTEIN

Protein includes the following: plant-based protein sources, fish and other seafood, poultry, eggs, cheese, red meat (beef, pork, veal, lamb), and game. For the purpose of managing prediabetes, it is recommended that you limit intake of red meat and game. You can choose to eat red meat two to three times per week at most, making sure to choose mostly lean meats. Plant-based proteins like tofu, beans, lentils, and edamame are lean and rich in fiber and usually contain very small amounts of saturated fats. As a result, they are great choices for your plate. If you eat animal protein, seafood should be eaten at least two times per week. Fish and seafood are rich in healthy omega-3 fats, which were shown to be good for metabolic health in a 2018 study on prediabetes and fish consumption. Seafood is also a good source of vitamin D, which tends to be low in people with prediabetes and was shown to lower the risk of progression to diabetes in a 2014 study published by the Endocrine Society. Chicken and turkey, mostly lean cuts, may also be included in your plate.

¼ PLATE = HEALTHY STARCH

Healthy whole-grain starches and starchy vegetables help keep you full and satisfied after a meal and should make up a quarter of your plate. There is no need to eliminate them completely from your diet. In fact, healthy starches provide energy to fuel your body and brain, and fiber needed for optimal digestion. A few examples of healthy whole grains include rice, 100 percent whole-wheat bread, whole-grain pasta, bulgur, oatmeal, quinoa, barley, and millet. Starchy vegetables including green peas, potatoes, sweet potatoes, corn, pumpkin, and plantains count as starches and are excellent choices, since they are high in vitamins, minerals, and fiber.

HEALTHY FAT COMPONENT

Foods that are rich in monounsaturated and polyunsaturated fats can be part of a healthy diet. Monounsaturated fats include avocado and avocado oil, canola oil, nuts (almonds, cashews, and pecans), olive oil and olives, peanut butter and peanut oil, sesame oil, and safflower oil. Polyunsaturated fats include omega-3–rich foods like walnuts, flaxseed and flaxseed oil, chia seeds, salmon, sardines, herring, mackerel, and tuna and omega-6–rich foods like tofu, eggs, peanut butter, sunflower seeds, sesame seeds, and pumpkin seeds.

Restock Your Pantry

You have the power to manage and even reverse prediabetes by making small, attainable changes to your diet. This begins with stocking your pantry with delicious, nutrient-rich foods. A diet high in saturated fat, salt, added sugar, artificial sweeteners, refined carbohydrates, and ultra-processed foods increases the risk of developing diabetes. Instead, increase your intake of nutrient-rich foods and eat mindful portions. These are the keys to managing and reversing prediabetes. Together we will explore easy ways to set up a pantry and refrigerator filled with nutrient-rich foods, making it easy and fun to make healthier food choices.

SHOP FOR GROCERIES WITH A PLAN

The first step for success is to organize, clean, and restock your pantry. In order to make shopping quick and easy, it is important for you to know what foods you already have on hand. As you organize your pantry, make sure to throw out products that are expired. If you wish to get rid of products that you no longer need or enjoy but that are still good to eat, donate them to a food pantry. Once your pantry is organized, you can use the Foods to Enjoy list provided in this chapter to restock your pantry.

Here's how to get started:

- Write a list of ingredients (old-fashioned paper or apps both work) based on the recipes you've planned for the week. If you can't find a particular ingredient, don't be afraid to substitute a similar ingredient. For instance, if a recipe calls for kale but your grocery store only has spinach, it is okay to swap kale for spinach.
- Check your refrigerator and pantry before shopping to make sure you don't buy unnecessary items. Make sure to refresh pantry staples that you want to always have handy.
- Focus on the outer perimeter of the grocery store. This usually includes the fresh produce, dairy, and protein sections. However, many healthy items can be found in the middle aisles, such as canned and frozen vegetables and beans with no added salt.
- Set a dedicated time for grocery shopping. Some people prefer to do all their shopping for the week on one day, while others prefer to go a couple of times per week.
- Make sure that you are not super hungry when you shop, since this may cause you to buy processed convenience foods that you don't truly need.
- Beware of misleading claims that falsely advertise highly processed foods as healthy. The following claims made on food packages do not mean that a food will support your health: fat-free, low-fat, low-calorie, sugar-free, no added sugar, light, lite, diet, all-natural.
- If you shop online, be aware of the advertisements that pop up on your screen. Be present while shopping online and don't be

influenced into buying highly processed food that may be falsely advertised as healthy.

- If you choose to indulge in buying desserts, chips, and other processed foods, do so mindfully. If you want to eat a cookie, buy a cookie made with high-quality ingredients.

HOW TO READ A NUTRITION LABEL

Learning how to read nutrition labels is a crucial part of making health-supportive food choices and purchasing nutrient-dense foods. Here are the steps that will help you read and understand food labels:

1. Start by reading the serving information at the top of the label. Pay close attention to the number of servings in a package or container and the size of a single serving. Remember that the label provides the calorie and nutrient information for one serving, not for the entire package or container.

2. Limit intake of foods that contain excessive amounts of added sugar, artificial sweeteners, sodium (salt), saturated fat, and trans fat. Compare similar products to each other to figure out which alternative is more health supportive.

3. Check the fiber content of the foods you are purchasing. You want to purchase products that are a good source of fiber. A good rule of thumb is to look for food products that contain around 5 grams or more of fiber per serving.

4. Purchase foods that provide the micronutrients (vitamins and minerals) your body needs to thrive. Look for foods that contain antioxidant-rich vitamins like vitamins A, C, D, K, and E, which play a role in diabetes management. If you are a vegan, make sure to eat foods fortified with vitamin B_{12}. Examples of vegan foods rich in vitamin B_{12} include fortified plant-based milks and yogurts and fortified nutritional yeast. Other important nutrients include iron, magnesium, potassium, and calcium.

5. Learn how to interpret percent daily values (%DV). The %DV tells you what percentage of the daily recommended amount of each nutrient a single serving of food contains. If your goal is to reduce

added sugar, sodium, or saturated fat, choose foods that contain 5 percent or less daily value of added sugar, salt, or saturated fat. If your goal is to increase your intake of a nutrient (like fiber, vitamins, and minerals), choose foods that contain 20 percent or higher DV of the nutrient you are trying to increase.

SERVING SIZES FOR COMMON FOODS

It can be helpful—and eye-opening—to be aware of the portions you eat. Here are some serving size guidelines to follow:

EQUIVALENT		FOOD	CALORIES
FIST	¾ cup	Rice Pasta Potatoes	150 150 150
PALM	4 ounces	Lean meat Fish Poultry	160 160 160
HANDFUL	1 ounce	Nuts Raisins	170 85
THUMB	1 ounce	Peanut butter Hard cheese	170 100

Foods to Enjoy

NOURISHING VEGETABLES

- Asparagus
- Beets
- Bell peppers
- Broccoli
- Butternut squash
- Carrots
- Cauliflower
- Celery
- Cucumber
- Jicama
- Leafy greens
- Leeks
- Mushrooms
- Onions
- Parsnips
- Radishes
- Sprouts
- Squashes
- Sweet peas
- Sweet potatoes
- Turnips
- Zucchini

EVERYDAY FRUIT STAPLES

- Apple
- Avocado
- Bananas
- Berries
- Lemons/limes
- Mangos
- Oranges/mandarins
- Pineapple

GRAINS

- Barley
- Brown rice (gluten-free)
- Oats (gluten-free)
- Quinoa (gluten-free)
- Rye
- Wild rice (gluten-free)

PLANT-BASED MILKS (NO SUGAR ADDED) AND DAIRY

- Almond milk
- Coconut milk
- Cow's milk (organic if possible)
- Plain yogurt (organic if possible)
- Rice milk
- Soy milk

BEANS AND LEGUMES

- ○ All beans
- ○ Chickpeas
- ○ Edamame
- ○ Fresh sprouts (your choice)

- ○ Lentils
- ○ Lima beans
- ○ Tempeh
- ○ Tofu

ANIMAL-BASED PROTEIN

- ○ Chicken/turkey (organic, cage-free; limit to 2 or 3 servings per week)
- ○ Eggs (organic, cage-free, or pasture-raised when possible)

- ○ Fish and shellfish (organic, wild-caught when possible)
- ○ Red meat (organic, pasture-raised; limit to 2 or fewer servings per week)

Foods to Limit or Eat in Moderation

In order to practice happy, mindful eating, it is important for you to understand that there is room at the table for all foods. Our goal is not to eliminate or prohibit any food group. Instead, we are striving to learn about the foods that should be consumed using more mindful portions. Foods that are high in added sugars, no-calorie sweeteners, saturated fats, and sodium should be limited. Many foods that may be marketed as healthy (flavored yogurt, granola, cereal, instant oatmeal, canned soup, and salad dressing) may contain hidden sugars. A good goal is to consume no more than 6 teaspoons (25 grams) of added sugar per day. Only 7 to 10 percent of your daily calories should come from saturated fats, and you should consume no more than 2,300 milligrams (mg) of sodium per day. Remember that foods that contain 5 percent DV or less of saturated fats, sodium, and added sugars are good choices.

FOODS TO EAT IN MODERATION

- Added sweeteners (honey, white sugar, maple syrup, agave, and molasses)
- Artificial no-calorie sweeteners
- Butter
- Deep-fried foods
- Desserts
- Fast food

FOODS TO LIMIT OR AVOID

- Energy drinks, soda, and sports drinks (diet and regular)
- Fatty cuts of red meat
- Juice cocktail
- Partially hydrogenated oils
- Processed meats
- Sweetened coffee and tea drinks

Staying on Track When Dining Out

My recommendation when dining out is to try not to stress about it! Remember that eating is a cultural and social tradition that connects us to friends, family, and our community. Here are some practical tips for dining out and practicing happy eating:

- Focus on starting your meal with vegetable options including salad, crudités, and vegetable platters.
- Aim to follow the My Plate: Prediabetes Reversal Method by including non-starchy vegetables (half your plate), healthy fats, protein, and whole grains or starchy vegetables while eating out.
- If you'd like to enjoy some refined carbohydrates (white bread, pasta), aim to make this only about a quarter of your plate. However, if you just really want to eat a pasta dish at an Italian restaurant once in a while, I encourage you to eat it without any guilt or stress.
- If you want dessert, get one for the table and share it.

Five Tips for Nutrition Success

1 **Embrace the practice of happy eating.**
Practice focusing your attention on all the new and delicious foods you will be adding to your plate instead of focusing on restricting your food intake. A great way to focus your attention on the foods you will be adding to your plate is by food journaling. Write down the foods you eat through-out the day and record how you feel before, during, and after meals.

2 **There's room at the table for all foods.**
You don't need to feel guilty about eating des-serts, carbohydrates, or any other food group. Managing prediabetes is about learning to eat mindful portions of all foods. Practice portioning out snacks and meals instead of mindlessly eating from the box, jar, or bag. Portioning your meals and snacks beforehand will allow you to achieve bal-anced nutrition and help you tune into your hunger and fullness cues.

3 **Plan ahead to create a balanced plate.**
The key to managing prediabetes is to create a balanced plate by making sure that half your plate is filled with non-starchy vegetables, a quarter is filled with whole-grain carbohydrates, and a quarter is filled with lean protein, with an added sprinkle of healthy fats and a serving of fruit. Setting up a meal plan, planning grocery shop-ping, and batch cooking will allow you to prep, cook, and pack your meals efficiently and with-out stress.

Choose wisely and mindfully when to eat or drink added sugar. Limit intake of added sugars by swapping sodas, energy drinks, and sweetened iced teas for unsweetened seltzer, herbal teas, green or black teas, or water infused with berries or herbs. It's more satisfying to enjoy a slice of cake, a few pancakes, or some ice cream than to mindlessly drink sweetened beverages that will not necessarily satisfy your appetite or hunger.

Be kind to yourself. Health is about practice, not perfection. Stressing yourself out about a meal plan or exercise routine will undermine your ability to reach your health goals, and it can have negative effects on your overall health, including your blood sugar levels. Try practicing mindfulness and meditation, and also treat yourself with loving-kindness and patience in order to reduce stress and find daily joy.

SOURCE: CDC T2 PREVENTION GUIDE

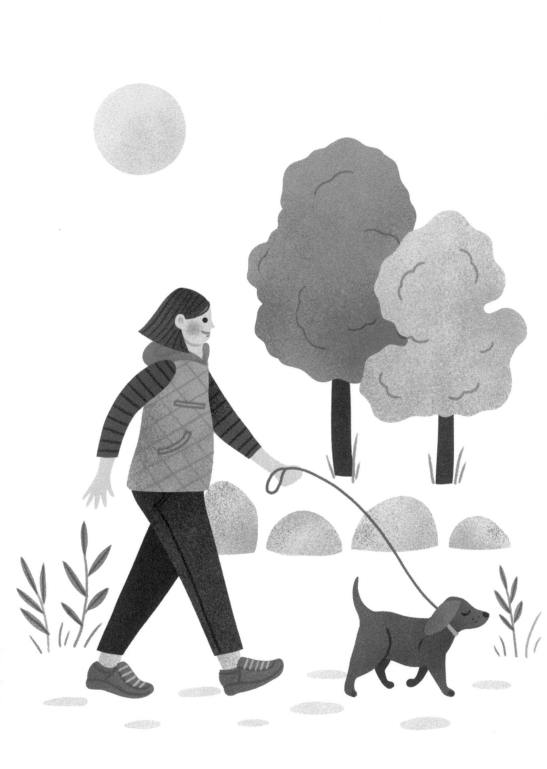

CHAPTER 3

Physical Activity and Prediabetes

R egular physical activity is essential for reversing prediabetes and preventing diabetes. In this chapter, you'll learn about the science behind the benefits of physical activity. I will also provide you with a physical activity routine that has specifically been developed to motivate you to move your body, manage insulin resistance, and reclaim your health.

How Physical Activity Helps

In 2010, the American College of Sports Medicine (ACSM) and the American Diabetes Association (ADA) released a joint statement expressing the critical role of routine physical activity that includes a mixture of aerobic (cardio) and resistance (strength) training in reversing prediabetes, delaying or preventing the onset of diabetes, and improving blood glucose control. In addition to being beneficial for glycemic (blood sugar) health, regular physical activity is linked to improved lipids (cholesterol and triglycerides), blood pressure, and cardiovascular health. The benefits of exercise can be instantly seen even after just one workout. A 2015 study published in *Diabetes Spectrum* by the ADA demonstrated that diabetic patients have increased insulin sensitivity (their body uses insulin more effectively) and improved glycemic control for 48 hours after just one exercise session. It is estimated that physical activity can improve the body's use of insulin for up to 72 hours after exercise.

The ACSM and the ADA recommend that people with diabetes or prediabetes, especially those who have a sedentary lifestyle, regularly engage in low to moderate physical activity that increases the heart rate. If you eat well but don't move your body and practice stress reduction techniques, you'll be undermining your efforts.

The greatest benefits from exercising are achieved through a combination of resistance training and aerobic exercises. Gentler types of exercise like restorative yoga or tai chi may also improve blood glucose balance. According to Harvard Health, exercise is also linked to better quality of life, improved sense of well-being, and reduction of depression symptoms. Studies in people who suffer depression show that participants of all age groups report fewer depression symptoms after exercising for long or short durations. Moving your body can improve your psychological well-being by allowing you to feel a sense of self-efficacy, self-mastery, and self-love. After exercising, levels of stress hormones like cortisol and adrenaline drop while levels of neurotransmitters like endorphins and serotonin increase. These neurotransmitters contribute to improving your mood, relaxation, sleep quality, and positive emotions.

How Much to Move Your Body

Physical activity recommendations are generally based on a person's current level of fitness, health history, and personal preferences. Aim to move your body on a daily basis and set the goal of achieving 150 minutes of moderate-intensity aerobic physical activity each week. Depending on your fitness level, you can also choose to do 75 minutes per week of vigorous-intensity aerobic physical activity. For strength training or resistance training, pencil it into your workout schedule two or three days each week, resting a day in between strength training sessions.

Build a Physical Activity Routine

Any physical activity is the perfect way to move your body and achieve your weekly fitness goals. You don't need to feel pressured to work out intensely or spend hours at the gym. The goal of this physical activity routine is to meet you where you are. Whether you are a person who hasn't worked out in a few years, a person who enjoys gentle movement like walks and restorative yoga, or a fitness lover who runs or bikes miles each week, this physical activity plan can be modified to meet your needs. Physical activity is a practice that requires patience and dedication. Although you may feel intimidated and sore at first, stick to your goal. Moving your body will undoubtedly uplift your mind, improve your quality of life, and restore your health.

CARDIO

Cardio, or aerobic physical activity, is exercise that increases the heart rate, such as cycling, dancing, swimming, fast-paced walking, and jogging. Studies suggest that aerobic training can help reverse metabolic syndrome, which includes a cluster of cardiovascular and metabolic conditions such as elevated blood pressure, high triglycerides and cholesterol, and excess accumulation of adipose fat around the organs. Participating in aerobic exercise also diminishes spikes of blood sugar after eating. Your goal is to increase aerobic fitness, since poor aerobic fitness is associated with high risk of health complications and mortality. Aerobic activities especially, and all exercise in general, reduce levels of triglycerides and cellular damage.

STRENGTH

Strength or resistance training, also known as anaerobic exercise, includes physical activities that use free weights, resistance, bands, weight machines, and medicine balls. For this exercise routine, you will use your own body weight to do a quick and safe strengthening routine.

Recent research shows that resistance training is therapeutic, effective for managing chronic diseases, and safe for elderly people and individuals who do not regularly exercise. Doing resistance training increases muscle mass and strengthens muscles. When you are doing a resistance training routine, it is important to focus on both the number of repetitions and the intensity of the exercise. In order to have a successful strength training routine, follow the progressive overload technique, which requires you to gradually increase repetitions and intensity as your fitness level increases.

A study published in the journal *Diabetes Care* found that high blood glucose levels may lead to loss of musculoskeletal mass and muscle atrophy. Some of the health benefits of resistance training include enhanced muscle strength, bone mineral density, and lean body mass as well as improved insulin sensitivity and glycemic control. According to the ADA, for those with prediabetes, participating in strength training exercise can result in lower fasting blood glucose levels up to 24 hours after exercising.

Use the following guidelines for your resistance training sets. Be sure to allow 30 to 45 seconds of rest between sets.

- Three sets of five reps (beginner)
- Three sets of eight reps (intermediate)
- Three sets of 10 reps (advanced)

Exercise 1: Plank (Modify for fitness level)

Start on your hands and knees with shoulders over elbows. Step the feet back one at the time and engage the glutes and thighs to keep the legs straight. Feet should be hip-width apart or wider. The body should form 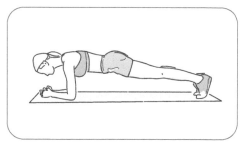 a straight line from shoulders to hips to heels. Think about pushing the ground away from you and pulling the belly button up toward the spine to keep the back flat. This exercise can be done on the floor or standing up using the wall for support.

Modification: Stand two feet from the wall on your tiptoes. Rest your elbows, forearms, and hands on the wall. Close your hands into a fist, making sure that elbows are under shoulders. Engage your abdomen by making sure that the buttocks are not sticking out and the back is curved. Hold this position for 30 to 60 seconds. Repeat three to five times and take 30 to 45 seconds to recover in between sets.

Exercise 2: Push-up (Modify for fitness level)

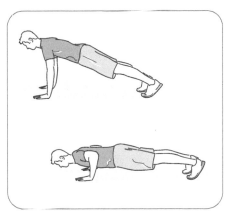

Place a mat on the floor and slowly lower your body to a horizontal position. Put the palms of your hands on the floor shoulder-width apart. Line your feet up with your shoulders and lift yourself off the mat.

Begin to lower your body by bending your elbows. Your body should be parallel to the ground when performing the push-up. Remember to breath out through your mouth and contract your abdominal muscles during each push-up movement. Slowly return to the starting position. Perform three sets of five and take 45 seconds to recover in between sets.

Modification: Instead of being on your toes in the starting position, place your knees on the mat and cross your ankles.

Exercise 3: Squat (Modify for fitness level)

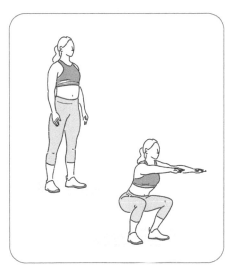

In a standing position, keep your chest up and make sure that hips, knees, and feet are shoulder-width apart. Keep both arms in a downward vertical position. Slowly begin to bend knees to a sitting position and raise arms into a horizontal position close to your chest. As you begin to bend your knees, remember to breathe out through your mouth and contract your abdominal muscles. Slowly return to the starting position and repeat. Perform three sets of five and take 45 seconds to recover in between sets.

Modification: Perform the squat using a chair as a guide and support.

Exercise 4: Side Lunge (Modify for fitness level)

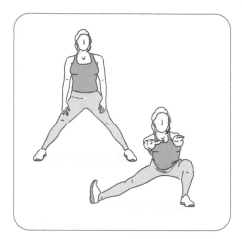

Start in a wide stance, with your feet wider than shoulder-width apart. Keep your back straight and shoulders relaxed by rolling them up, back, and down. Engage the core by making sure you are not sticking out your buttocks or tucking them in. Look forward at a point in front you and keep your chin in a stable, neutral position.

Shift your weight to your right leg, sitting your hips back and bending your right knee to about 90 degrees while your left leg goes straight. Push up from your right leg, driving your weight through your heels, back to the starting position. Repeat the exercise on your left side. This completes one rep. Perform three sets of five reps and take 45 seconds to recover in between sets.

Modification: To make lunges more accessible, limit your range of motion (less than a 90-degree bend) or stand next to a wall and lightly rest your hand on the wall for support.

Exercise 5: Arm circles

Stand with your feet hip-width apart. Lengthen your back, relax your shoulders (roll shoulders up, back, and down), and engage the core. Slowly raise your arms to shoulder height, making sure that they are parallel to the floor. Do not hyperextend the elbows, but have a gentle bend in them. Slowly rotate your arms forward, making small circles. Complete five forward-moving circles.

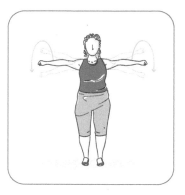

Then rotate your arms backward, making small circles. Complete five backward-moving circles. This completes one set. Slowly lower your arms. Perform three sets of five reps and take 45 seconds to recover in between sets. To make this exercise more challenging, hold 1- or 2-pound weights.

Exercise 6: Mountain Climbers (Modify for fitness level)

Start in the plank position. Bring your right knee up toward your chest. Return to the starting position and then bring your left knee up toward your chest. This completes one rep. Perform three sets of five reps and take 45 seconds to recover in between sets.

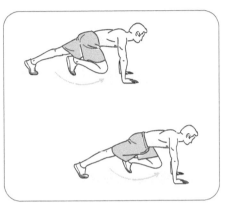

Modification: Stand with your hands behind the nape of the neck, making sure to support your head. Spread your elbows apart. Bring your right knee up toward your chest. Switch sides. Bring your left knee up toward your chest.

Exercise 7: Jumping Jacks (Modify for fitness level)

Start with your feet together and hands at your sides. Jump both your feet outside your shoulders while also raising your arms over your head, bringing the hands close together. Jump your feet back together while bringing your hands down and landing in the starting position. This completes one rep. Perform three sets of 10 reps and take 45 seconds to recover in between sets.

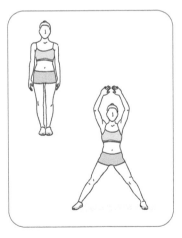

Modification: For a lower impact move, step-tap the feet outward while raising the arms to replace the jumping movement.

Five Tips for Exercise Success

1 **Be optimistic about your new fitness routine, but set realistic goals.** If you are new to working out, setting unrealistic and extreme fitness goals can make you feel defeated, stressed, and burned out. Moving your body is a practice that takes time, patience, and self-kindness.

2 **Keep moving all day, especially on days that you may not have time for a workout.** Moving your body throughout the day will help you achieve your goal of 150 minutes of physical activity per week. Try to get steps any chance you get. If you are meeting a friend for coffee, take the coffee to go and enjoy a walk in the park or around the neighborhood. Set up walking meetings at work and pencil in walk or stretch breaks during the workday. Take a walk after dinner to relax, use the stairs instead of the elevator, and park farther away from the store to get in a few more steps.

3 **Be fearless and let go of feelings of embarrassment or negative thoughts about your body.** I often hear from clients that they won't exercise because they are uncomfortable or embarrassed about exercising in public or in front of friends and family. Most people who go to the gym, dance classes, martial arts classes, or yoga classes are there with the same purpose as you: to embrace a healthier lifestyle. Everyone at one point or another is a beginner, and you should not be embarrassed if you can't easily do all the exercises at first. Keep practicing. Appreciate your body, embrace its current fitness state, and be kind to yourself.

 Listen to your body when you are unwell or tired. If you are sleep deprived or have not eaten and hydrated, it is okay if you do not work out. Pushing yourself to exercise when you are exhausted or unwell can make you feel sick, cause injury, or lead to prolonged recovery. If you are sick, it is best to rest.

Hydration is key to prediabetes management and a productive and safe exercise routine. Fluid intake should be a daily habit practiced consistently. Buy a reusable water bottle and carry it around with you all day, aiming to refill your water bottle several times each day. Be aware of signs of dehydration like dark urine and thirst. Keep in mind that when you are sweating due to heat or physical activity, you will need to drink more water. Although hydration recommendations vary from person to person, generally men should aim to drink about 3 liters (13 cups) of fluid per day and women should drink about 2.2 liters (10 cups) of fluid each day. Although beverages like coffee, tea, juice, and milk count toward your fluid intake goal, you should aim to drink mostly water. Spice up your water by adding citrus, mint, basil, cilantro, dill, rosemary, or berries, or try drinking sodium-free, sweetener-free sparkling water.

CHAPTER 4

Mental Health, Sleep, and Prediabetes

E mbracing a health-supportive lifestyle allows you to focus on nurturing your physical, mental, and emotional well-being and happiness. By embracing a lifestyle philosophy that prioritizes and champions your overall well-being, it is possible to reverse and manage prediabetes. The building blocks for improving mental health, managing stress, and sleeping better are to improve your nutrition status through happy and mindful eating and increase physical activity through mindful movement and enjoyable exercise or recreation. In this chapter, you will explore the roles that nurturing your mental health, reducing stress, and getting good-quality sleep play in reversing prediabetes and optimizing health.

Mental Health

Taking care of your mind is just as important to your health as taking care of your body. A crucial part of managing and reversing prediabetes is to understand the mind–body connection and prioritize caring for your physical, emotional, spiritual, and mental health needs. Dealing with conditions like chronic stress, depression, and trauma may increase your risk of developing type 2 diabetes, so it is important to assess your mental health with honesty and kindness. While it is normal to feel stress or sadness, if you are coping with chronic anxiety, depression, or an eating disorder, make sure to seek support from a mental health professional or your primary care physician as soon as possible.

After receiving a prediabetes diagnosis, you may feel overwhelmed, sad, angry, and anxious about the need to change your eating and lifestyle habits and the possibility of developing diabetes. This is normal, but it is important to begin to shift your focus to cultivating compassion, forgiveness, and gratitude in addition to nurturing hope and optimism about the future. Self-reflection is a valuable tool to learn from our past experiences and behaviors, but it is important not to linger in the past. Mindfulness encourages us to focus our attention on the present moment by letting go of guilt and regret for our past emotions. Focusing on the present moment will allow you to realize that you are capable of achieving your highest health goals, improving your quality of life, and maximizing your happiness.

DEVELOP A POSITIVE MINDSET

Developing a positive mindset allows you to approach successes and challenges with optimism and an upbeat outlook. In order to develop a positive mindset, it is important to believe in your own self-efficacy and trust in your ability to make beneficial decisions and long-term behavioral changes. Having a positive mindset does not mean that you don't ever feel negative emotions or that you avoid and ignore challenging situations; instead, it means that you focus on making the best of the challenges that you must confront. For instance, you may feel discouraged or disappointed to learn that you have insulin resistance. These emotions are valid. However, instead of focusing on feeling guilty or bad about yourself, you can practice shifting your focus to being grateful that you are in a position where it is still possible to reverse prediabetes and prevent full-blown diabetes. Furthermore, you can perceive this as an opportunity to set time aside for self-care and loving-kindness toward yourself. A positive mindset will allow you to develop and nurture character traits that will help you succeed in achieving your health goals. These positive traits include:

Optimism. Trusting in your abilities and committing to your efforts to make positive behavior changes. Optimism also helps you let go of negative expectations.

Acceptance. Learning to accept that health is about practice, not perfection. The only thing that this book asks is that you make an honest effort to improve your well-being and that you show up for yourself patiently and lovingly.

Resiliency. Accepting that you will not be perfect or always successful and trusting in your ability to learn from your mistakes and bounce back from adversity without lingering in negative emotions.

FIND YOUR MOTIVATION

In order to find motivation, it is important to explore your intention for making lifestyle changes. What is your intention for adding more vegetables and fruits to your diet? For instance, you may want to add more vegetables and fruits to your plate because you want to improve your blood glucose level. Perhaps you'd like to move your body more because you want to lead a healthier life that allows you to spend more quality time with your family. Keeping an intention present will allow you to find the motivation needed to make positive lifestyle changes. Embracing the GROW (Goals, Reality, Options, Will to Do) model may help you feel motivated.

Goals: Define the most important changes and objectives you want to achieve.

It is important to set short- and long-term goals that are realistic and attainable. What specific goals do you want to focus on? How does this goal align with your vision for the present and future? How will it feel and look when you achieve your goals?

_____

_____

_____

_____

_____

_____

_____

Reality: Clearly identify the obstacles that may impede or slow down progress and analyze the current reality of the situation.

What internal and external obstacles will you need to overcome? Who can support you in overcoming obstacles?

_____

_____

_____

_____

_____

_____

_____

Options: Discover and understand what different options are available to reach your goals.

What are some different ways you can achieve your goals? What will happen if you don't follow through on taking actions to achieve your goals? What are some of the benefits of adopting practices that help you reach your goals?

_____

_____

_____

_____

_____

_____

_____

_____

Will to Do: Affirm your commitment to take action and decide what actions you will take.

Specify what actions/steps you will take to achieve your goals. How, when, and where will you implement these actions/steps? How will you track your progress?

_____

_____

_____

_____

_____

_____

_____

_____

CELEBRATE YOUR VICTORIES

Celebrating your achievements and your commitment to making positive lifestyle changes is key to feeling happy and motivated. It is important to acknowledge small wins on a daily basis. Remember that achieving small goals over time will lead to great improvements in your long-term health. Small wins can include making sure that you follow the **My Plate: Prediabetes Reversal Method** at most meals or go for a 30-minute walk after work three times per week. Over time, through a series of small wins, you may achieve a big goal like reducing your blood glucose levels or A1C. Finding the time and space to celebrate your everyday victories is a form of self-love and self-care. Writing your goals is the perfect way to visualize and celebrate your victories. At the end of this chapter, you will find a journal prompt that will help you keep track of your goals and serve as a reminder to celebrate your achievements.

FIND NONFOOD COMFORTS AND REWARDS

As previously mentioned, there is no shame in craving or eating comforting food after a difficult day or indulging in cake during a celebration. However, it is also important to explore other ways to sustainably feed our feelings. If you turn to food as your main source of comfort and then feel guilty or ashamed after, this creates a negative cycle. It is important to learn how to recognize the difference between physical hunger and emotional hunger. Physical hunger emerges gradually, usually hours after eating a meal, and it is satisfied after you feel full from eating a meal. Emotional hunger usually emerges suddenly and doesn't coincide with mealtimes. Furthermore, it is not satisfied after eating and may lead to feelings of guilt and shame.

Mindless eating occurs when you eat without paying attention to your hunger and fullness cues and without savoring the food you are ingesting. Learning what may trigger mindless and/or emotional eating is important to improving your overall well-being. For instance, do you eat mindlessly when you're tired or after a night of poor sleep? Do you eat emotionally when you are stressed or sad? Findother nonfood-related comforts, rewards, or activities. Some examples include calling a loved one who is supportive, playing with your pet, going for a walk, dancing to your favorite song, reading a book, spending time in nature, trying a new physical activity or class, taking a relaxing bath, watching your favorite movies, reading a new book, and learning a new skill or hobby.

DON'T BE AFRAID TO ASK FOR HELP

Having a support system to turn to is helpful for reaching your goals and improving your sense of well-being. Ask friends or members of your family to support your dietary and lifestyle changes. It is important to realize that asking for help or support does not mean you are not capable of reaching your goals on your own or that you are a burden to others. This book is a complete guide to empowering you to achieve your goals. However, if you feel like you are struggling with your mental health, I encourage you to reach out to your primary care physician, psychologist, psychiatrist, or other trusted health professional. If you need additional support for making dietary changes, find an integrative registered dietitian nutritionist (IntegrativeRD.org). It may also be helpful to set up a few sessions with a physical therapist, exercise physiologist, or certified personal trainer to create a physical activity routine that meets your fitness level and goals.

Stress Management

When a person is confronted with stress, the body releases cortisol, one of the hormones responsible for the fight-or-flight response. Cortisol signals the body to stop insulin production and raises blood glucose levels in order to increase the amount of energy available for immediate use by the body. Suffering from chronic stress due to work schedules, relationships, or a demanding lifestyle may cause the body to constantly produce cortisol, which may lead to high blood glucose levels and increased appetite. People who suffer from chronic stress may turn to emotional eating for stress relief and comfort. It is perfectly normal and healthy to eat food when you are happy or celebrating or to occasionally indulge in your favorite food as a pick-me-up after a difficult day. Emotional eating becomes a concern when eating is your main coping mechanism for stress. Stress can make it more challenging to make positive decisions and adopt health-supportive lifestyle changes like feeling motivated to exercise or meal prep.

PRACTICE ACCEPTANCE AND COMMIT TO SELF-DISCOVERY

Instead of attempting to control or ignore uncomfortable feelings and thoughts, it may be healing to accept and experience them. It is important to identify negative emotions and realize that you are not defined by them. By exploring your thoughts and emotions, you may be able to more clearly identify your personal values and goals and take the steps necessary to fulfill those goals. Furthermore, you may be able to develop better ways to think about and respond to negative emotions.

IMPLEMENT EMOTION-FOCUSED COPING

Emotion-focused coping asks you to find ways to navigate negative emotions or feelings when confronted with a challenging situation. Instead of trying to change the challenging situation, emotion-focused coping strategies encourage a person to find ways to relax or deal with a stressful situation through various behaviors and exercises. These include meditation, breathing exercises, relaxation techniques, positive reframing of negative emotions, finding time to spend on your own to restore your energy, and seeking social support, including from health professionals. Emotion-focused coping is particularly important for managing a challenging situation that one may not be able to alter.

IMPLEMENT PROBLEM-FOCUSED COPING

Problem-focused coping strategies require a person to confront a problem or stressor in an attempt to resolve it or make it better. For example, a way to relieve stress after getting a prediabetes diagnosis is to take actions like adding more vegetables to your diet or going on a walk to increase physical activity. Taking action to resolve issues that are within reach is a way to promote peace of mind and a sense of well-being.

Sleep

Sleep is essential to health. While you are sleeping, your body and mind rest and recharge. Proper sleep is necessary for proper brain function, hormonal balance, heart and circulatory health, repair of tissues, and immunity. Poor sleep quality is linked to greater risk of prediabetes. A 2016 study published in *Current Diabetes Reports* found that people who sleep less than six hours per night are more likely to have higher fasting glucose levels and increased risk of developing diabetes. Lack of sleep may also lead to hormonal disturbances and irregular eating patterns. For instance, when you do not get enough sleep, the levels of ghrelin, the hormone responsible for making you feel hungry, increase, while the levels of leptin, the hormone that signals fullness, decrease. As a result, you may feel hungrier when you don't get enough good-quality sleep. Prioritizing sleep should be a nonnegotiable aspect of your wellness routine.

CREATE A NIGHTLY ROUTINE

Sleep experts, including those at Harvard Health, recommend creating a relaxing nightly routine in order to de-stress and decompress before bedtime. Stress and anxiety often interfere with good sleep. Some rituals that you may enjoy as a part of your bedtime routine include meditating, practicing a breathing exercise, giving yourself an oil massage, taking a warm bath, journaling, or reading your favorite book. Feeling relaxed before bedtime may help you fall asleep faster. Setting up a relaxing bedtime routine does not require a huge time commitment. If you are able to consistently set aside 10 to 15 minutes to do a relaxing and enjoyable activity before bedtime, you will find that you get better sleep and feel more refreshed to tackle the next day.

GET AT LEAST SEVEN TO EIGHT HOURS OF SLEEP PER NIGHT

As previously mentioned, getting less than six hours of sleep has been linked to increased risk of developing diabetes. There is no one-size-fits-all approach to sleep. Some people may need more or less sleep, so it is important to determine how much sleep you need for optimal health. As you get older, you may need less sleep. However, it is important to make an effort to get the amount of sleep you need to feel refreshed, clear-minded, and energetic. A good way to know if you're getting enough sleep is to closely monitor how long it takes you to fall asleep. If you struggle to fall asleep for more than 15 minutes, you may be getting too much sleep, or it may be related to stress or excess caffeine. If you are so exhausted and sleepy that you fall asleep immediately, it may mean that you are not sleeping enough. It is important to adjust your sleep schedule based on your preferences and schedule demands to make sure that you are getting enough sleep. If you need to wake up early to get to work on time, then you may need to have an earlier bedtime to reach your sleep goal. However, if you struggle to fall asleep at an early bedtime, then perhaps moving your bedtime back a couple of hours may be helpful.

WORK WITH YOUR CIRCADIAN RHYTHMS

Circadian rhythms are a group of 24-hour body processes responsible for regulating the sleep/wake cycle, an internal clock that lets you know when it is time to sleep and when it is time to wake up. Some signs that your circadian rhythm is off-balance include struggling to fall asleep or to wake up. Circadian rhythms also play a role in digestion and hormone regulation. It is important to understand that our circadian rhythms are affected by our genetics and lifestyle. For example, some people are naturally early birds who feel most energized in the early morning, while others are night owls who feel more productive in the evening or at night. The sleep/wake cycle is significantly influenced by light exposure (both sun and artificial light), caffeine consumption, stress, jet lag, and irregular bedtime routines. By maintaining a consistent sleep schedule throughout the week, including on weekends and holidays, you'll help maintain the body's internal clock. This will help you fall asleep faster, wake up at the same time every day, and feel more energized in the morning.

KEEP IT COOL

Room temperature affects sleep onset and quality. Sleeping in a room that is too warm can affect the body's ability to regulate its temperature and reach the needed sleep cycles to restore the body and mind. This can lead to fatigue, discomfort, and restlessness while sleeping. Sleeping in a cool room is one of the most important things you can do to get a good night's sleep. For the most revitalizing sleep, aim to sleep in a room that is 60 to 67 degrees Fahrenheit (15.6 to 19.4 degrees Celsius). Taking a shower or bath before bed may help your body relax and cool down before you go to sleep.

Five Tips for Mental Health and Sleep Success

TIP 1: Just Breathe. Deep breathing can help relieve stress and anxiety. It allows for full oxygen exchange, which can help reduce your heartbeat and blood pressure. To begin, follow these simple steps:

1. Find a comfortable seat or position. (You can sit on a chair, the floor, or a meditation cushion or lie down on a bed or the floor.)

2. Close your eyes and be still. (Try to stop fidgeting or moving around.)

3. Inhale deeply and slowly through your nose. Exhale deeply and slowly through your mouth. Repeat three times.

4. Go back to your regular breathing pattern and slowly begin to focus your attention on the inhale and exhale.

5. Notice every inhale and exhale. On the inhale you can silently repeat to yourself "let," and on the exhale you can silently repeat to yourself "go." With each inhale and exhale you let go of stress, tension, and judgment. If your mind wanders away from focusing on your breathing, it's okay! Just bring back your attention to each inhale and exhale. You can do this for a few breaths, several minutes, or as long as you enjoy it.

TIP 2: Meditate. Meditation is a powerful practice that you can seamlessly incorporate into your daily life. It has been shown to help people reduce stress, manage anxiety, nurture well-being, and improve their sleep and cognitive function. Studies have also linked meditation to reduced blood pressure, pain control, and addiction management.

TIP 3: Set Electronics Boundaries. Being constantly plugged into your phone, tablet, or laptop may cause stress and keep you from truly enjoying the present moment. Exposure to blue light before bed interferes with your sleep/wake cycle. Make sure to set guidelines around electronics use. Making time to disconnect from technology, especially right before bedtime, may also help you find time to reconnect with yourself and your loved ones.

TIP 4: Rest and Relaxation Are Nonnegotiable. Rest and relaxation are key to nurturing your physical, mental, and emotional well-being. While there is still some social stigma around prioritizing mental health and acknowledging when you are struggling mentally or emotionally, it is important to remember that mental health is just as important as physical health. There is no shame in setting boundaries regarding your work schedule or social commitments if it will help you prioritize your sleep and mental wellness.

TIP 5: Health Is a Practice, Not Perfection. Show up for yourself every day to the best of your ability. Some days you may successfully reach all your daily health goals, and other days you may find it impossible to reach even one. It's okay if you are not perfect! No one is. Be kind and patient with yourself.

part II

Meal Plan and Recipes

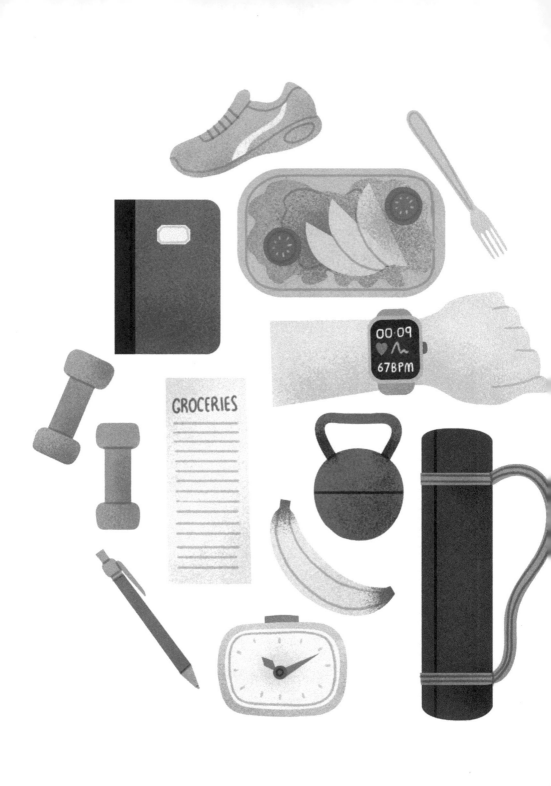

CHAPTER 5

Putting It All Together: A Two-Week Plan

Now that you have all the tools needed to take charge of your health, nurture your well-being, and reverse prediabetes, it's time to implement these tools into your daily routine. I encourage you to remember that health is not about perfection, it's a practice. It is important to trust in your growing knowledge, self-efficacy, and dedication to improving your health. In the next two weeks, you will develop and practice the skills that will allow you to reverse and manage prediabetes.

About the Plan

The goal of this two-week plan is to provide you with the support and guidance you need as you learn to eat, move, and relax in ways that work for your medical needs and food preferences. This book is not meant as a restrictive or fad diet but as a helpful guide filled with information, meal plans, recipes, mindfulness practices, and fitness routines to innovate your lifestyle and reverse prediabetes. The weekly shopping lists and meal plans will help you streamline your nutrition and develop your new cooking routine, and the habit tracker will help you monitor the changes you're making in every aspect of your life.

As you make changes, you may feel overwhelmed or hesitant. It is completely normal and understandable to feel stressed when making changes, even positive ones. Whenever you feel overwhelmed, I'd like you to remember that you should be immensely proud of yourself for taking an active role in your health. It takes courage to make lifestyle changes and to reflect on how to improve your own well-being.

I encourage you to follow the two-week plan to the best of your ability. It was created in a flexible way that allows for your input and creativity. I also encourage you to engage in journaling as an exercise to learn more about yourself and explore which of these health practices will work for your body, lifestyle, culture, budget, and food preferences.

Week 1 Shopping List

PANTRY

- All-purpose flour
- Allspice, ground
- Almonds, slivered
- Apple cider vinegar
- Baking powder
- Baking soda
- Balsamic vinegar
- Basil, dried
- Bay leaves
- Black pepper, freshly ground
- Bulgur
- Cardamom, ground
- Cayenne pepper
- Chia seeds
- Cinnamon, ground
- Coconut sugar (or white or raw)
- Dark brown sugar
- Extra-virgin olive oil or avocado oil
- Flaxseed, ground
- Granola bar (less than 8 grams added sugar)
- Hemp seeds
- Honey
- Nutmeg, ground
- Oats, steel-cut, old-fashioned, or quick
- Oregano, dried
- Paprika, smoked
- Paprika, sweet
- Peanut butter, crunchy or smooth
- Peanuts, roughly chopped
- Pecans, roughly chopped
- Pitas, whole wheat
- Pumpkin seeds, roasted
- Raisins
- Red pepper flakes
- Rosemary, dried
- Salt
- Sea salt

- Sunflower seeds
- Thyme, dried
- Vanilla extract
- Walnuts

- Whole-wheat pastry flour
- Whole grains, cooked (quinoa, oats, rice)

CANNED/BOTTLED

- Beetroot, 1 (15-ounce) can
- Bread crumbs 1 (15-ounce) can
- Black beans, 2 (15-ounce) cans
- Capers 1 (3.5-ounce) bottle
- Chickpeas, 3 (15-ounce) cans
- Corn, 1 small can
- Crushed tomatoes, 1 (28-ounce) can
- Green olives, 2 (6-ounce) bottles

- Kalamata olives, 2 (6-ounce) bottles
- Lemon juice (1 tablespoon)
- Lime juice (1 small bottle)
- Maple syrup, 1 (32-ounce) bottle
- Roasted red bell peppers, 1 (16-ounce) jar
- Soy sauce (1 bottle)
- Tahini, 1 (16-ounce) jar
- Tomato paste (1 small can)
- Vegetable broth (2 quarts)

PRODUCE

- Apples, any variety (3) and Granny Smith (3)
- Arugula (4 cups)
- Avocado (1)
- Baby carrots, 1 (2-pound) bag
- Baby portobello mushrooms, sliced (20 ounces)
- Basil, fresh (2 bunches)
- Berries, any variety (1 pint)
- Celery (1 bunch)
- Cilantro, fresh (2 bunches)
- Cucumber (2 medium)
- Fennel bulb (1 medium)
- Garlic (2 bulbs)
- Ginger, fresh, 1 (1-inch piece)
- Green bell pepper (1 small)

- Honeydew melon (1)
- Kale (1 bunch)
- Kale, purple, chopped (1 bunch)
- Lemon (1)
- Limes (4)
- Mint, fresh (1 bunch)
- Onions (1 large, 2 medium, 2 small yellow, 1 small red)
- Oranges (4)
- Pear, any variety (1)
- Red Thai chile or jalapeño pepper (1)
- Scallions (1 bunch)
- Shallot (1)
- Spinach, fresh, 2 (16-ounce) bags

- Strawberries (1 pint)
- Tomato (1 medium and 2½ pounds, any variety)
- Veggie sticks, precut (2 servings)

DAIRY AND EGGS

- Cheddar cheese, grated, 1 (8-ounce) bag
- Cheese sticks (2)
- Eggs, 1 (dozen) carton
- Milk, dairy or plant-based, 1 (half-gallon) carton
- Yogurt, plain, dairy or vegan (2 cups)

PROTEINS

- Lean ground turkey, 1 (20-ounce) package
- Roasted chicken or canned organic roasted chicken breast, no added salt (2 cups)
- Shrimp, medium, peeled and deveined (3 pounds, 21 to 25 per pound)

FROZEN FOODS

- Edamame, 1 (16-ounce) bag
- Mango, 1 (16-ounce) bag
- Peaches, 1 (16-ounce) bag
- Pineapple, 1 (32-ounce) bag

	BREAKFAST	SNACK	LUNCH	SNACK	DINNER
DAY 1	Huevos Rancheros Muffins (page 81)	Green Apple Smoothie (page 75)	Orange Fennel Salad (page 91)	Beetroot Chickpea Hummus with fresh veggie sticks	Creole-Style Shrimp Étouffée (page 126) with Muffuletta Olive Salad (page 97)
DAY 2	Creamy Overnight Oats with Apple Pear Cinnamon Compote (page 78)	1 tablespoon peanut or almond butter and 1 medium apple	Roasted Tomato Soup (page 100)	*Leftover* Green Apple Smoothie	*Leftover* Creole-Style Shrimp Étouffée with Muffuletta Olive Salad
DAY 3	*Leftover* Huevos Rancheros Muffins	*Leftover* Beetroot Chickpea Hummus with veggie sticks	Lemon Mint Bulgur Salad (page 102)	1 granola bar (less than 8 grams added sugar)	*Leftover* Roasted Tomato Soup
DAY 4	*Leftover* Creamy Overnight Oats with Apple Pear Cinnamon Compote	1 cheese stick and 1 cup carrots	Massaged Kale and Strawberry Salad (page 88)	Gooey Peanut Butter Chocolate Cookies (page 142)	Meatball Pita Sandwich (page 127)
DAY 5	Mediterranean-Style Breakfast Bowl (page 82)	*Leftover* Gooey Peanut Butter Chocolate Cookies	*Leftover* Lemon Mint Bulgur Salad	1 tablespoon peanut butter and celery sticks	*Leftover* Massaged Kale and Strawberry Salad
DAY 6	Peach Mango Lassi (page 74)	1 cup no-sugar-added plain yogurt with 1 cup berries	Balsamic-Glazed Mushrooms and Chickpeas (page 136) with Honeydew Melon and Almond Gazpacho (page 137)	*Leftover* Gooey Peanut Butter Chocolate Cookies	*Leftover* Meatball Pita Sandwich
DAY 7	*Leftover* Mediterranean-Style Breakfast Bowl	1 cheese stick or ¼ cup almonds and 1 medium apple	Spicy Apple and Carrot Salad (page 96)	*Leftover* Peach Mango Lassi	*Leftover* Balsamic-Glazed Mushrooms and Chickpeas with Honeydew Melon and Almond Gazpacho

GOALS	DAY 1	DAY 2	DAY 3
VEGGIES *5+ servings per day*	☐ ☐ ☐ ☐ ☐	☐ ☐ ☐ ☐ ☐	☐ ☐ ☐ ☐ ☐
FRUITS *4+ servings per day*	☐ ☐ ☐	☐ ☐ ☐	☐ ☐ ☐
HEALTHY FATS *1 serving at every meal*	☐ ☐ ☐	☐ ☐	☐ ☐
PROTEIN *1 serving at every meal*	☐ ☐	☐	☐ ☐
WATER INTAKE *(aim for 1 ounce of water per pound of body weight)*			
MINDFULNESS PRACTICE *(deep breathing, meditation, gratitude prayer) 3 per day*	☐ ☐ ☐	☐ ☐	☐ ☐
MINDFUL MOVEMENT/ PHYSICAL ACTIVITY *150 minutes per week*	Activity Type: _____ *Duration:*	Activity Type: _____ *Duration:*	Activity Type: _____ *Duration:*
SLEEP *7 to 9 hours/day*	*Duration:*	*Duration:*	*Duration:*
DAILY INTENTION *What will you do to ensure success?*			
REFLECTIONS *How are you feeling about your progress?*			

DAY 4	DAY 5	DAY 6	DAY 7	WEEKLY TOTALS
Activity Type:	Activity Type:	Activity Type:	Activity Type:	
Duration:	Duration:	Duration:	Duration:	
Duration:	Duration:	Duration:	Duration:	

Week 2 Shopping List

PANTRY

- All-purpose flour
- Almond flour
- Almonds, raw or roasted
- Apple cider vinegar
- Baking powder
- Baking soda
- Bay leaves
- Black pepper, freshly ground
- Cardamom, ground
- Cashews, raw unsalted
- Celery salt
- Chia seeds
- Chipotle chili powder
- Chocolate chips
- Cinnamon, ground
- Coconut oil
- Coriander, ground
- Cumin, ground
- Dark brown sugar
- Extra-virgin olive oil
- Flaxseed, ground
- Garlic powder
- Granola bars (less than 8 grams added sugar)
- Honey
- Maple syrup
- Miso, white
- Nutmeg, ground
- Nuts, any variety
- Oat flour
- Olives
- Oregano, dried
- Paprika, smoked
- Pumpkin seeds, unsalted raw or roasted
- Raisins
- Red pepper flakes
- Salt
- Sea salt
- Sesame oil
- Sugar, white, coconut, or raw
- Thyme, dried
- Vanilla extract, pure
- Whole grains, cooked (white or brown rice, quinoa, millet, or barley)
- Whole-wheat pastry flour
- Whole-wheat penne
- Whole-wheat tortillas

CANNED/BOTTLED

- Apple juice, 1 (32-ounce) bottle
- Black beans, 1 (15-ounce) can
- Chickpeas, 1 (15.5-ounce) can
- Corn, 1 small can
- Crushed tomatoes, 1 (28-ounce) can
- Dijon mustard
- Navy beans, 1 (15.5-ounce) can

- ○ Pumpkin puree,
  1 (15-ounce) can
- ○ Red kidney beans,
  2 (15-ounce) cans
- ○ Roasted red bell pepper,
  1 (16-ounce) jar
- ○ Vegetable broth (3 quarts)

PRODUCE

- ○ Apples, any variety
  (2 medium), Granny Smith
  (2 medium)
- ○ Arugula (1 bunch)
- ○ Avocados (4)
- ○ Baby carrots, 3 (1-pound) bags
- ○ Balsamic vinegar
- ○ Bananas (2 medium)
- ○ Basil, fresh (1 bunch)
- ○ Bell peppers, any color (2),
  red (2)
- ○ Berries (1 pint)
- ○ Butter lettuce (3 heads)
- ○ Button mushrooms (3 pints)
- ○ Celery (1 bunch)
- ○ Cilantro (2 bunches)
- ○ Dill (1 bunch)
- ○ Garlic (2 bulbs)
- ○ Ginger, fresh, 1 (1-inch) piece
- ○ Jalapeño pepper (2)
- ○ Lemons (3)
- ○ Limes (3)
- ○ Mint (1 bunch)
- ○ Onions (5 medium,
  red or yellow,
  1 small red)
- ○ Oranges, seedless (3)
- ○ Raspberries, fresh or frozen
  (3 pints)
- ○ Salad greens,
  1 (16-ounce) bag
- ○ Scallions (1 bunch)
- ○ Shallots (2)
- ○ Spinach, fresh,
  1 (8-ounce) bags
- ○ Tomato (1 medium),
  cherry (5 pints)
- ○ Veggie sticks, precut
  (2 servings)
- ○ Yellow squash (1 medium)
- ○ Zucchini (2 medium)

DAIRY AND EGGS

- ○ Butter (1 stick)
- ○ Cheese sticks (2)
- ○ Eggs, 1 (half-dozen) carton
- ○ Milk, 1 (half-gallon) carton
- ○ Mozzarella cheese, fresh,
  1 (8-ounce) ball
- ○ Parmesan cheese, grated
  (¼ cup plus 2 teaspoons)
- ○ Yogurt, plain and no sugar
  added (2 cups)

PROTEINS

- ○ Extra-firm tofu (2 pounds)
- ○ Italian sausage (½ cup)
- ○ Silken tofu (1 cup)

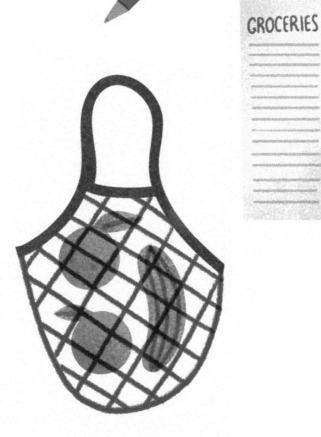

	BREAKFAST	SNACK	LUNCH	SNACK	DINNER
DAY 8	Pumpkin Spice Chia Seed Pudding (page 80)	¼ cup nuts (any variety) and 1 medium banana	*Leftover* Spicy Apple and Carrot Salad	Zesty Guacamole (page 132) with veggie sticks	New Orleans–Style Red Beans (page 116) with Farmers' Market Salad with Homemade Ranch Dressing (page 92)
DAY 9	Breakfast Burrito (page 84)	*Leftover* Zesty Guacamole with veggie sticks	Zucchini Basil Soup (page 103)	1 granola bar (less than 8 grams added sugar)	*Leftover* New Orleans–Style Red Beans with Farmers' Market Salad with Homemade Ranch Dressing
DAY 10	*Leftover* Pumpkin Spice Chia Seed Pudding	1 cup no-sugar-added plain yogurt with 1 cup berries	Mint Pesto Pasta Salad (page 94)	Raspberry Crumble Bars (page 140)	Vegetarian (or Not) Fajitas (page 124)
DAY 11	*Leftover* Breakfast Burrito	1 cheese stick and 1 medium apple (any variety)	*Leftover* Zucchini Basil Soup	*Leftover* Raspberry Crumble Bars	*Leftover* Mint Pesto Pasta Salad
DAY 12	Dutch Chocolate Chip Pancakes (page 83) with Raspberry Chia Seed Marmalade (page 140)	Creamy Orangesicle Smoothie (page 76)	Plant-Based Caesar Salad (page 90)	1 cup no-sugar-added plain yogurt with 1 cup berries	*Leftover* Vegetarian (or Not) Fajitas
DAY 13	*Leftover* Creamy Orangesicle Smoothie	¼ cup nuts and 1 medium apple	Vegetarian Chipotle Sesame Poke Bowl (page 120)	*Leftover* Raspberry Crumble Bars	Warming Ginger Carrot Bisque (page 106)
DAY 14	*Leftover* Dutch Chocolate Chip Pancakes with Raspberry Chia Seed Marmalade	1 granola bar (less than 8 grams added sugar)	*Leftover* Warming Ginger Carrot Bisque	1 cheese stick and 1 cup carrots	*Leftover* Vegetarian Chipotle Sesame Poke Bowl

GOALS	DAY 1	DAY 2	DAY 3
VEGGIES *5+ servings per day*	☐ ☐ ☐ ☐ ☐	☐ ☐ ☐ ☐ ☐	☐ ☐ ☐ ☐ ☐
FRUITS *4+ servings per day*	☐ ☐ ☐ ☐	☐ ☐ ☐ ☐	☐ ☐ ☐ ☐
HEALTHY FATS *1 serving at every meal*	☐ ☐ ☐	☐ ☐ ☐	☐ ☐ ☐
PROTEIN *1 serving at every meal*	☐ ☐ ☐	☐ ☐	☐ ☐
WATER INTAKE *(aim for 1 ounce of water per pound of body weight)*			
MINDFULNESS PRACTICE *(deep breathing, meditation, gratitude prayer) 3 per day*	☐ ☐ ☐	☐ ☐ ☐	☐ ☐ ☐
MINDFUL MOVEMENT/ PHYSICAL ACTIVITY *150 minutes per week*	Activity Type: ———— *Duration:*	Activity Type: ———— *Duration:*	Activity Type: ———— *Duration:*
SLEEP *7 to 9 hours/day*	*Duration:*	*Duration:*	*Duration:*
DAILY INTENTION *What will you do to ensure success?*			
REFLECTIONS *How are you feeling about your progress?*			

DAY 4	DAY 5	DAY 6	DAY 7	WEEKLY TOTALS
Activity Type:	Activity Type:	Activity Type:	Activity Type:	
Duration:	Duration:	Duration:	Duration:	
Duration:	Duration:	Duration:	Duration:	

After the Plan

Congratulations on taking charge of your health! I am very proud of your commitment to prioritize your well-being, and I am grateful for your dedication. In the past couple of weeks, you've learned and practiced the skills needed to successfully achieve your health goals. This plan was created with the goal of empowering you to reverse prediabetes, but it can also serve as a guide for you and your loved ones to nurture balanced nutrition and a health-supportive lifestyle.

As we've previously discussed, health is a practice that you commit to everyday. I encourage you to take the skills you've developed through this book and continue to use them in your daily health journey. Whenever you feel like you need a refresher, more structure, or added support, remember that this book is always here for you. I trust in your ability to lead a healthier lifestyle and to improve your relationship with food, your loved ones, and yourself.

Five Tips for Long-Term Success

1 **Don't sweat the small stuff!** Remember that adopting a healthy lifestyle is not about being perfect all the time. It is a practice that varies from day to day. If you are unable to eat a balanced meal one day, it is not the end of the world, and if you can't make it to the gym because you are working late, there is no need to feel guilty.

2 **Your self-worth is not based on your weight, health status, or physical appearance.** The most important thing you can do for your own health is to practice loving-kindness toward yourself and others.

3 **You can eat all foods.** Make an effort to stop moralizing food. Food is neither good nor bad. It is just food. Therefore, feeling guilty after eating a rich or decadent food is counterproductive.

4 **Commit to your new lifestyle.** Ditch the restrictive, fad diet approach and embrace a health-supportive lifestyle that meets your needs and is sustainable. Play around with tips and techniques and make it your own.

5 **Practice mindfulness when you cook, meditate, or work out.** Paying close attention to the present moment can help you learn about yourself and your tendencies. Staying focused in the present moment can also greatly reduce stress, as it prevents you from thinking about the past or the future.

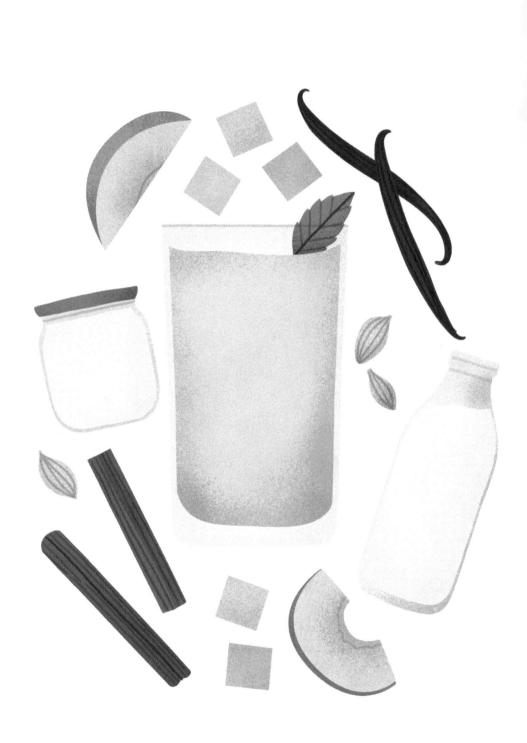

CHAPTER 6

Breakfasts and Smoothies

Peach Mango Lassi

SERVES 4 | PREP TIME: 10 MINUTES

30 MINUTES OR LESS ▪ **DAIRY-FREE** ▪ **GLUTEN-FREE** ▪
NUT-FREE ▪ **VEGAN** ▪ **VEGETARIAN**

I was inspired to add lassi to my own diet after I visited Kerala in India. This refreshing and lightly spiced drink is the perfect mixture of natural sweetness, a bit of tartness, and some warming spices. Both peaches and mangos are excellent sources of vitamins and minerals and have a low glycemic index. Low glycemic index fruits do not cause a rise in blood sugar, especially when paired with a healthy protein like yogurt.

1½ cups frozen peaches
1 cup frozen mango
1 cup plain dairy or vegan yogurt
1 cup milk (dairy or plant-based)

1 teaspoon ground cinnamon
¼ teaspoon ground cardamom
1 teaspoon vanilla extract

1. In a blender, blend the peaches, mango, yogurt, milk, cinnamon, cardamom, and vanilla until smooth.
2. Serve immediately or pour into airtight jars for storage. The lassi will remain fresh for up to 3 days in the refrigerator.

Ingredient Tip: A lassi is a traditional Indian yogurt drink that can be spiced up with rose water, cardamom, ginger, cinnamon, and other warming spices. In addition to spices, you can add a variety of fruits and herbs, like mint and spearmint, to your lassi.

Per Serving: Calories: 120; Carbohydrates: 18g; Fat: 4g; Saturated Fat: 2g; Sugars: 17g; Cholesterol: 13mg; Protein: 5g; Fiber: 2g; Sodium: 57mg

Green Apple Smoothie

SERVES 4 | PREP TIME: 10 MINUTES

30 MINUTES OR LESS • DAIRY-FREE • GLUTEN-FREE • VEGAN •
VEGETARIAN

Who says you can't kick-start your morning with veggies? This creamy
and zesty smoothie is filled with heart-healthy fats and fiber that
promote healthy cholesterol levels thanks to chia seeds and avocado.
Ginger's gentle spiciness wakes up the senses while helping promote a
healthy digestive system and balanced blood sugar.

1 Granny Smith apple, cored
and chopped

2 cups frozen pineapple

2 tablespoons avocado

2 cups milk (dairy or plant-based)

2 teaspoons chia seeds

2 cups fresh spinach or
1 cup frozen spinach

1 tablespoon grated ginger (about a
1-inch piece ginger root)

1. In a blender, blend the chopped apple, pineapple, avocado, milk,
   chia seeds, spinach, and ginger until smooth.
2. Serve immediately or pour into airtight jars for storage. The smoothie
   will remain fresh for 2 to 3 days in the refrigerator.

Substitution Tip: Replace the spinach with any other greens that you
enjoy. Kale also works great in this smoothie.

Per Serving: Calories: 153; Carbohydrates: 25g; Fat: 4g; Saturated Fat: 2g; Sugars: 18g;
Cholesterol: 10mg; Protein: 6g; Fiber: 4g; Sodium: 71mg

Creamy Orangesicle Smoothie

SERVES 4 | PREP TIME: 10 MINUTES

30 MINUTES OR LESS · DAIRY-FREE · GLUTEN-FREE · VEGAN ·
VEGETARIAN

A walk down memory lane inspired the creation of this smoothie, which
is reminiscent of the classic orange ice-cream pops I enjoyed every
summer as a child. This version is much healthier. Oranges, raspberries, and carrots are excellent sources of immune support with plenty of
vitamins A and C. Pumpkin seeds are high in magnesium, which is linked
to improved blood sugar balance.

2 seedless oranges, peeled and
   sectioned
1 cup fresh or frozen raspberries
1 cup water
½ cup yellow squash chunks

¼ cup raw unsalted pumpkin seeds
¼ teaspoon ground cinnamon
2 teaspoons vanilla extract
3 dates, pitted (optional)

1. In a blender, blend the oranges, raspberries, water, squash, pumpkin
   seeds, cinnamon, vanilla, and dates (if using) until smooth.
2. Serve immediately or pour into airtight jars for storage. The smoothie
   will remain fresh for up to 3 days in the refrigerator.

Substitution Tip: This smoothie recipe works well with other citrus
fruits like blood oranges and clementines. You can also swap the
raspberries for any of your favorite berries.

Per Serving: Calories: 104; Carbohydrates: 14g; Fat: 4g; Saturated Fat: 1g; Sugars: 8g;
Cholesterol: 0mg; Protein: 4g; Fiber: 4g; Sodium: 3mg

Protein-Rich Granola

SERVES 4 | PREP TIME: 10 MINUTES | COOK TIME: 20 MINUTES

30 MINUTES OR LESS • **DAIRY-FREE** • **GLUTEN-FREE** • **VEGAN** • **VEGETARIAN**

This crunchy homemade granola is low in added sugar and rich in seeds and nuts, which provide healthy protein and fat for optimal nutrition and balanced blood sugar. Make a couple of batches of this granola and store in airtight glass jars for up to 3 months. Simply combine with yogurt or milk and fresh berries for the perfect quick breakfast or snack.

2 cups plain rolled oats or gluten-free oats
½ cup pumpkin seeds or sunflower seeds
½ cup pecans
¼ cup almonds
¼ cup raisins

2 teaspoons pumpkin pie spice
½ teaspoon salt
2 tablespoons extra-virgin olive oil
½ teaspoon vanilla extract
2 tablespoons honey
2 tablespoons maple syrup

1. Preheat the oven to 350°F. Line an 13-by-18-inch baking sheet with parchment paper and set aside.
2. In a large bowl, mix the rolled oats, seeds, pecans, almonds, raisins, pumpkin spice, and salt until thoroughly combined.
3. Drizzle the olive oil, vanilla, honey, and maple syrup over the oat mixture and use a spatula or wooden spoon to stir until well coated.
4. Place the mixture on the prepared baking sheet.
5. Bake for 20 minutes, making sure to stir occasionally.

Ingredient Tip: If you are gluten intolerant or suffer from celiac disease, make sure to purchase oats labeled gluten-free. You can use any type of nuts, seeds, or no-sugar-added dried fruit like cherries and cranberries to change up the recipe.

Per Serving: Calories: 581; Carbohydrates: 63g; Fat: 33g; Saturated Fat: 3g; Sugars: 22g; Cholesterol: 0mg; Protein: 13g; Fiber: 8g; Sodium: 296mg

Creamy Overnight Oats with Apple Pear Cinnamon Compote

SERVES 4 | PREP TIME: 15 MINUTES, PLUS OVERNIGHT TO CHILL
COOK TIME: 10 MINUTES

DAIRY-FREE · GLUTEN-FREE · VEGAN · VEGETARIAN

The comforting smell of cinnamon, apples, and oatmeal in morning warms my heart. It reminds me of the oatmeal that my dad prepared for me every day before I headed to school. In a perfect world, we would all have time in the morning to eat a slow breakfast, but life is hectic. I created this recipe as a way for you to be able to have a quick and easy breakfast that is also comforting, nourishing, and delicious. If you make this recipe before going to bed, when you wake up you will have the perfect bowl of creamy, ready-to-eat oats in the refrigerator.

For the compote

½ teaspoon extra-virgin olive oil

⅓ cup roughly chopped pecans

2 tablespoons raisins

1 Bosc, Anjou, or Bartlett pear, peeled and cut into ½-inch dice

1 Honeycrisp, Granny Smith, or Golden Delicious apple, peeled and cut into ½-inch dice

½ teaspoon ground cinnamon

¼ teaspoon ground nutmeg (optional)

¼ teaspoon ground allspice (optional)

1 teaspoon honey

½ teaspoon vanilla extract

¼ cup water

For the oats

1 cup steel-cut, old-fashioned, or quick oats

2 cups milk (plant-based or dairy)

½ teaspoon vanilla extract

½ teaspoon ground cinnamon (optional)

2 tablespoons chia seeds

1 tablespoon hemp seeds

To make the compote

1. In a large skillet, heat the oil over medium heat. Add the pecans and toast for 1 minute.
2. Add the raisins, pears, apples, cinnamon, nutmeg, and allspice. Sauté for about 2 minutes until the spices become fragrant.
3. Add the honey, vanilla, and water, gently stirring.
4. Cook uncovered for 5 to 7 minutes over medium heat until the fruit is tender and some of the liquid is absorbed.

To make the oats

5. In a large jar or airtight container, combine the oats, milk, vanilla, cinnamon (if using), chia seeds, and hemp seeds. Shake or stir to combine.
6. Place in the refrigerator and let sit overnight. In the morning, the oats will be creamy and ready to eat. You can add more milk to the oats if they absorb too much milk overnight.
7. Stir in the compote and enjoy.

Variation Tip: If you are craving warm oatmeal, add more milk to the overnight oats and heat the mixture in the microwave for about 1 minute or in a small saucepan until warm. Top with 1 cup of fresh fruit (½ cup of berries and ½ sliced banana) or 1 medium whole fruit sliced or diced (mango, peach, pear, or apple all work great). Drizzle with honey or maple syrup (1 to 2 teaspoons at most) or add a few pieces of dried fruit for a touch of sweetness. You could also add up to 2 teaspoons of peanut butter or almond butter for more protein.

Per Serving: Calories: 337; Carbohydrates: 45g; Fat: 14g; Saturated Fat: 2g; Sugars: 20g; Cholesterol: 10mg; Protein: 9g; Fiber: 8g; Sodium: 60mg

Pumpkin Spice Chia Seed Pudding

SERVES 4 | PREP TIME: 15 MINUTES, PLUS 2 TO 3 HOURS OR OVERNIGHT TO CHILL

DAIRY-FREE · GLUTEN-FREE · ONE POT · VEGAN · VEGETARIAN

Pumpkin spice is a warming and naturally sweet blend that will enhance your chia seed pudding and turn it into a decadent breakfast. Pumpkin is an excellent source of vitamin A and beta-carotene. Beta-carotene is linked to numerous health benefits including a strong immune system and improved heart, eye, and skin health. Furthermore, a diet rich in pumpkin has been linked to lower risk of developing metabolic syndrome and poor blood sugar control.

1 cup chia seeds
4 cups milk (dairy or plant-based)
1 teaspoon ground cinnamon
½ teaspoon ground nutmeg
¼ teaspoon ground cardamom
 (optional)

1 teaspoon vanilla extract
1 cup unsweetened canned
 pumpkin puree
¼ cup raisins
2 tablespoons maple syrup

1. In a glass jar or airtight container, combine the chia seeds, milk, cinnamon, nutmeg, cardamom (if using), vanilla, pumpkin puree, raisins, and maple syrup. Shake or stir to combine.
2. Refrigerate overnight or for at least 2 to 3 hours before eating.

Ingredient Tip: Top with 1 cup of berries and 2 teaspoons of peanut or almond butter for added protein and fiber. You can prepare this pudding the night before to have it ready in the morning.

Per Serving: Calories: 478; Carbohydrates: 55g; Fat: 23g; Saturated Fat: 5g; Sugars: 26g; Cholesterol: 20mg; Protein: 18g; Fiber: 22g; Sodium: 129mg

Huevos Rancheros Muffins

SERVES 4 | PREP TIME: 15 MINUTES | COOK TIME: 20 MINUTES

DAIRY-FREE · GLUTEN-FREE · VEGETARIAN

Mornings are hectic, and it's not always easy to eat a filling and nourishing breakfast. There is no excuse to skip breakfast anymore with this recipe. I was inspired to create these egg muffins after eating a mini quiche at my favorite Latin-inspired coffee shop in New York City. I like to make these on the weekend and store the leftovers in the refrigerator for the perfect on-the-go breakfast. Rich in protein and fiber, these muffins will satisfy your craving for a savory, quick, and nutritious breakfast.

Extra-virgin olive oil, for greasing (optional)

6 eggs

½ teaspoon dried oregano

¼ teaspoon smoked paprika

¼ teaspoon salt

2 tablespoons canned corn kernels, drained and rinsed

3 tablespoons canned black beans, drained and rinsed

2 tablespoons chopped fresh cilantro

¼ cup grated cheddar cheese (optional)

1. Preheat the oven to 375°F. For easier cleanup, line a muffin tin with paper liners; otherwise, grease the muffin tin with oil.
2. In a medium bowl, whisk the eggs, oregano, paprika, and salt.
3. Stir in the corn, black beans, cilantro, and cheddar cheese (if using).
4. Using a ¼-cup measure, distribute the mixture into the muffin tin. Bake until each muffin is set in the center, 18 to 20 minutes.
5. Serve warm, at room temperature, or cool. Make sure to refrigerate leftovers. Leftovers will last 3 to 4 days in the refrigerator.

Technique Tip: Bake these muffins in a reusable BPA-free silicone muffin tin for a more eco-friendly option.

Per Serving: Calories: 123; Carbohydrates: 3g; Fat: 7g; Saturated Fat: 2g; Sugars: 0g; Cholesterol: 279mg; Protein: 10g; Fiber: 1g; Sodium: 253mg

Mediterranean-Style Breakfast Bowl

SERVES 4 | PREP TIME: 15 MINUTES | COOK TIME: 20 MINUTES

DAIRY-FREE • VEGAN • VEGETARIAN

Starting out the morning with veggies can seem like an unrealistic goal. However, I am here to tell you that adding veggies to your morning routine doesn't need to be difficult. This bowl is gushing with rustic vegetables, legumes, and fragrant herbs that will elevate your morning routine and make you feel excited about eating veggies for breakfast.

2 teaspoons extra-virgin olive oil

4 ounces baby portobello mushrooms, sliced

1 teaspoon smoked paprika

1 medium tomato, diced

1 (15.5-ounce) can chickpeas

1 cup chopped purple kale

1 cup chopped spinach

1½ tablespoons balsamic vinegar

2 teaspoons dried oregano

1 tablespoon chopped fresh basil

½ teaspoon salt

1 cup cooked whole grains (quinoa, oats, rice)

1 sunny-side-up, fried, hard-boiled, or scrambled egg

¼ cup grated Parmesan cheese (optional)

1. In a medium skillet, heat the oil over medium heat.
2. Add the mushrooms and paprika and sauté until tender and aromatic, 7 to 10 minutes.
3. Add the tomato and chickpeas and sauté for 3 minutes more.
4. Add the kale, spinach, balsamic vinegar, oregano, basil, and salt. Cook until the greens are wilted but not soggy, 3 to 5 minutes.
5. To assemble the bowl, place your choice of cooked whole grain in the bowl, then ladle a generous scoop of the Mediterranean mushroom and chickpea mixture over it, and top with an egg and grated cheese (if using).

Per Serving: Calories: 197; Carbohydrates: 28g; Fat: 6g; Saturated Fat: 1g; Sugars: 5g; Cholesterol: 47mg; Protein: 9g; Fiber: 6g; Sodium: 444mg

Dutch Chocolate Chip Pancakes

MAKES 12 PANCAKES | PREP TIME: 15 MINUTES
COOK TIME: 20 MINUTES

DAIRY-FREE • NUT-FREE • VEGAN • VEGETARIAN

Whip these pancakes up for a weekend brunch or make a batch of batter and store it in the refrigerator for up to 5 days. Use the recipe for Raspberry Chia Seed Marmalade (page 140) for a delicious topping.

1 tablespoon extra-virgin olive oil, plus more for greasing
3 tablespoons ground flaxseed
1 cup, plus 1 tablespoon warm water
1 cup whole-wheat flour
½ cup oat flour
2 teaspoons baking powder
¼ teaspoon baking soda

1 teaspoon cinnamon (optional)
¼ teaspoon salt
1 cup milk (dairy or plant-based)
4 teaspoons apple cider or white vinegar
2 tablespoons honey
¼ cup chocolate chips
1 banana, cut into rounds (optional)

1. Preheat the oven to 400°F. Line a 9-inch round cake pan with parchment paper and grease with olive oil.
2. In a small bowl, whisk together the flaxseed and warm water. Set aside.
3. In a large bowl, whisk together the whole-wheat flour, oat flour, baking powder, baking soda, cinnamon (if using), and salt.
4. In a separate bowl, whisk together the milk, vinegar, honey, and 1 tablespoon of oil.
5. Pour the flaxseed mixture and the liquid ingredients into the dry ingredients. Combine using a rubber spatula or whisk, making sure not to overmix. Gently fold in the chocolate chips.
6. Pour the batter into the cake pan. Place the banana slices (if using) on top of the wet batter.
7. Bake for 15 to 17 minutes or until you insert a toothpick into the pancake and it comes out clean and the bananas are caramelized.

Per Serving (2 pancakes): Calories: 225; Carbohydrates: 33g; Fat: 8g; Saturated Fat: 3g; Sugars: 10g; Cholesterol: 4mg; Protein: 6g; Fiber: 5g; Sodium: 177mg

Breakfast Burrito

SERVES 4 | PREP TIME: 15 MINUTES | COOK TIME: 20 MINUTES

DAIRY-FREE • VEGETARIAN

One of my all-time favorite comfort foods is the humble burrito. I love to eat these burritos for breakfast, lunch, and dinner, since they are quick to make and easy to pack to take on the go. The spicy and savory ingredients native to communities in Mexico and Southwest United States inspired this recipe. Filled with mushrooms, shallots, and black beans, this burrito provides fiber and prebiotics crucial for balanced blood sugar and a healthy digestive system.

For the burrito

2 teaspoons extra-virgin olive oil

1 cup mushrooms, diced

1 shallot or onion, diced

1 medium tomato, diced

1 teaspoon dried oregano

½ teaspoon smoked paprika

2 tablespoons canned corn kernels, drained and rinsed

2 tablespoons canned black beans, drained and rinsed

4 whole-wheat tortillas

For the scrambled eggs (optional)

3 or 4 eggs

1 tablespoon milk

Salt

Freshly ground black pepper

2 teaspoons butter

To make the burrito

1. In a medium skillet, heat the oil over medium heat.
2. Add the mushrooms and shallot to the skillet and cook until tender and aromatic, about 7 minutes.
3. Add the tomato, oregano, and paprika and sauté for 3 minutes.
4. Add the corn and black beans and cook until warm and tender, about 10 minutes. Stir frequently.

5. To assemble the burrito, heat the tortillas in a skillet or microwave for about 1 minute.
6. Stuff each tortilla with the burrito filling and scrambled eggs (if using).

To make the scrambled eggs (optional)

7. Break the eggs into a small bowl, adding a splash of milk if you like, and beat until they are well blended. Season with salt and pepper to taste.
8. Heat the butter in a small nonstick sauté pan over low heat.
9. When the butter is hot, add the egg mixture. Cook over low heat, making sure to stir occasionally with a spatula. Cook until the eggs are soft, moist, and set but not browned. Remove from heat and add to the burritos.

Variation Tip: If you'd like to make this burrito vegan, replace the eggs with tofu, seitan, or tempeh. Simply add your choice of vegan protein to the skillet during step 3 and continue to follow the recipe method as instructed. You can also add your choice of animal protein including 2 cups of ground chicken, turkey, or ground beef. Add the animal protein during step 3 and continue to follow the recipe method as instructed.

Per Serving: Calories: 173; Carbohydrates: 30g; Fat: 5g; Saturated Fat: 1g; Sugars: 5g; Cholesterol: 0mg; Protein: 6g; Fiber: 4g; Sodium: 163mg

CHAPTER 7

Salads and Light Mains

Massaged Kale and Strawberry Salad

SERVES 4 | PREP TIME: 20 MINUTES

**30 MINUTES OR LESS · DAIRY-FREE · GLUTEN-FREE ·
NUT-FREE · VEGAN · VEGETARIAN**

Adding fruit to your salads can truly brighten and elevate them. The natural tanginess of the strawberries complements the earthy flavor of kale. Furthermore, the vitamin C found in strawberries helps with the absorption of iron found in kale. In this recipe, feel free to use lacinato kale, green curled kale, or purple curled kale. The goal of massaging kale is to make it more tender to chew and easier to digest. Massaging the kale also helps the vinaigrette flavor and coat the kale leaves more fully.

For the vinaigrette

2 cups strawberries (about 15 strawberries)

2 teaspoons extra-virgin olive oil

2 teaspoons maple syrup

1 tablespoon lemon or lime zest (optional)

½ teaspoon lemon or lime juice

1 teaspoon balsamic vinegar

½ teaspoon salt

For the salad

1 head kale (about 7 cups), washed and stemmed

¼ teaspoon salt

1 teaspoon apple cider vinegar (or vinegar of choice)

1 teaspoon extra-virgin olive oil

½ cup strawberries, sliced

½ cup roasted pumpkin seeds

To make the vinaigrette

1. In a blender, blend the strawberries, oil, maple syrup, lemon zest (if using), lemon juice, balsamic vinegar, and salt and blend until smooth and creamy.

To make the salad

2. Using your hands, tear the kale into bite-size pieces and place in a large bowl. Add the salt, apple cider vinegar, and oil.

3. Using your hands, massage the kale until it is tender and slightly wilted, about 3 minutes.
4. Drizzle the strawberry balsamic vinaigrette over the massaged kale and toss until the kale is well coated.
5. Sprinkle the sliced strawberries and pumpkin seeds over the salad to finish.

Storage Tip: This recipe makes about 1 cup of vinaigrette. Place leftovers in an airtight container or jar and save it to dress other salads or vegetables during the week. It remains fresh in the refrigerator for 4 to 5 days.

Ingredient Tip: You can substitute kale with spinach, arugula, lettuce, or watercress and toss in your favorite protein (tofu, chicken, sliced egg) to make this a complete meal.

Per Serving: Calories: 120; Carbohydrates: 7g; Fat: 9g; Saturated Fat: 1g; Sugars: 3g; Cholesterol: 0mg; Protein: 6g; Fiber: 2g; Sodium: 211mg

Plant-Based Caesar Salad

SERVES 4 | PREP TIME: 15 MINUTES

30 MINUTES OR LESS · DAIRY-FREE · NUT-FREE · VEGAN · VEGETARIAN

I've created a plant-based Caesar dressing that is decadent and creamy as well as naturally high in fiber and protein. I recommend that you make a batch of this dressing and use it to spice up sandwiches and wraps or as a dipping sauce for vegetables throughout the week.

For the dressing

1 cup silken tofu (about ½ block), drained

1 garlic clove, chopped

Juice of 1 lime (about 2 tablespoons)

1 tablespoon extra-virgin olive oil

1 tablespoon balsamic vinegar

1 tablespoon mild white miso

2 teaspoons soy sauce

1½ teaspoons honey

¼ teaspoon Dijon mustard (or mustard of choice)

For the salad

5 cups butter lettuce (or lettuce of choice), torn into bite-size pieces

1 pint cherry tomatoes or 2 Roma tomatoes, quartered

½ cup roasted pumpkin seeds

2 teaspoons Parmesan cheese (optional)

To make the dressing

1. In a blender, blend the tofu, garlic, lime juice, oil, vinegar, miso, soy sauce, honey, and mustard until creamy.

To make the salad

2. Mix the lettuce and tomatoes in a large bowl, and then drizzle with the dressing.

3. Sprinkle with the pumpkin seeds and Parmesan cheese (if using).

Per Serving: Calories: 197; Carbohydrates: 12g; Fat: 13g; Saturated Fat: 2g; Sugars: 6g; Cholesterol: 0mg; Protein: 11g; Fiber: 3g; Sodium: 358mg

Orange Fennel Salad

SERVES 4 | PREP TIME: 15 MINUTES

30 MINUTES OR LESS • DAIRY-FREE • GLUTEN-FREE • VEGAN • VEGETARIAN

Zesty orange and spicy fennel flavors marry in this salad to make the perfect combination that is traditionally served in Southern Italy as a refreshing side dish. Oranges and other citrus fruits are high in fiber and have a low glycemic index, making them excellent foods to help achieve balanced blood sugar. Fennel is a good source of fiber, potassium, magnesium, and calcium, all important nutrients for promoting heart health.

1 medium fennel bulb

3 oranges, plus 3 tablespoons orange juice

4 cups arugula

1 tablespoon balsamic vinegar

2 teaspoons extra-virgin olive oil

¾ teaspoon salt

½ cup green olives, pitted

½ cup walnuts or sliced almonds, roasted (optional)

1. Quarter the fennel bulb, making sure to remove the core. Cut the fennel into thin half-moons.
2. Peel the oranges completely. Use a knife to remove the orange pith and seeds (if the oranges are not seedless). Cut the oranges into bite-size segments or half-moons.
3. Place the fennel, orange segments, and arugula into a large bowl. Set aside.
4. In a small bowl, make a vinaigrette by whisking together the orange juice, vinegar, oil, and salt.
5. Drizzle the salad with the vinaigrette, and then sprinkle with the olives and walnuts (if using).

Time-Saving Tip: If you want to make prep faster, use unsweetened canned oranges.

Per Serving: Calories: 123; Carbohydrates: 21g; Fat: 4g; Saturated Fat: 1g; Sugars: 13g; Cholesterol: 0mg; Protein: 2g; Fiber: 5g; Sodium: 598mg

Farmers' Market Salad with Homemade Ranch Dressing

SERVES 4 | PREP TIME: 15 MINUTES | COOK TIME: 5 MINUTES

30 MINUTES OR LESS · DAIRY-FREE · GLUTEN-FREE · NUT-FREE · VEGAN · VEGETARIAN

Ranch dressing is rightfully one of the most popular dressings in the United States. Velvety, creamy, and tangy—who can resist it? I've created my own velvety ranch dressing using cashews, which have been linked to lower blood insulin levels and lower blood sugar.

For the dressing

½ cup raw unsalted cashews

¾ cup boiling water

2 teaspoons extra-virgin olive oil

1 shallot

1 garlic clove

2 tablespoons lemon juice

1 teaspoon salt

¼ teaspoon freshly ground black pepper

¼ teaspoon Dijon mustard (or mustard of choice) (optional)

For the salad

5 cups butter lettuce (or lettuce of choice), torn into bite-size pieces

2 cups spinach

1 pint cherry tomatoes, halved, or plum tomatoes, cut in ½-inch dice

1 (15.5-ounce) can chickpeas, drained and rinsed

½ ripe avocado, diced (optional)

1 tablespoon fresh dill, roughly chopped (optional)

To make the dressing

1. Soak the cashews in the boiling water that has been taken off the heat for at least 5 minutes while you prepare the rest of the ingredients.
2. In a small sauté pan, heat the oil over low heat. Once the oil is hot, add the shallot and garlic, cooking until fragrant and lightly browned, about 5 minutes. Remove from heat.

3. In a blender, blend the cashews with the soaking water, the sautéed shallot and garlic, and the lemon juice, salt, pepper, and mustard until the dressing is creamy.

To make the salad

4. Place the lettuce, spinach, tomatoes, chickpeas, and avocado (if using) in a bowl and top with the dressing. Toss to combine and garnish with the dill (if using).

Substitution Tip: You can swap the chickpeas for 1 cup of roasted chicken or turkey. If you are allergic to cashews or don't have them handy, you can substitute them with ½ cup of plain regular or Greek yogurt.

Per Serving: Calories: 230; Carbohydrates: 25g; Fat: 12g; Saturated Fat: 2g; Sugars: 7g; Cholesterol: 0mg; Protein: 9g; Fiber: 6g; Sodium: 628mg

Mint Pesto Pasta Salad

SERVES 4 | PREP TIME: 20 MINUTES | COOK TIME: 20 MINUTES

DAIRY-FREE · VEGETARIAN

Pasta can be part of your prediabetes-friendly diet and health-supportive eating philosophy. The key to eating carbohydrates like pasta is to pair them with healthy fats, vegetables, and protein. This creamy pesto salad is the perfect make-ahead dish. I recommend making a batch of it on the weekend and storing it in your refrigerator. It is the perfect go-to lunch or quick dinner after a busy day. The longer the pasta marinates in the pesto, the more flavorful it becomes.

For the pesto

½ cup almonds, raw or roasted
½ cup pumpkin seeds,
   raw or roasted
1 garlic clove
3 cups spinach

2 cups mint leaves
¼ cup extra-virgin olive oil
2 tablespoons lemon juice
1 tablespoon mild white miso

For the pasta salad

5 cups whole-wheat penne
   (or pasta of choice)
2 cups spinach
1 cup arugula
1 cup cherry tomatoes, halved
½ cup chopped roasted
   bell peppers

¼ cup olives, pitted and roughly
   chopped or whole
½ teaspoon salt
½ cup fresh mozzarella cheese, cut
   into bite-size pieces
¼ cup Parmesan cheese (optional)

To make the pesto

1. In a food processor, pulse the almonds, pumpkin seeds, garlic, spinach, mint, oil, lemon juice, and miso. Process until smooth.

To make the pasta salad

2. Cook the pasta according to the package directions.
3. In a large bowl, toss together the cooked pasta, spinach, arugula, tomatoes, peppers, olives, and salt.
4. Add ½ cup of pesto, making sure to coat all the pasta and vegetables.
5. Top with the fresh mozzarella and sprinkle with the Parmesan (if using).

Substitution Tip: You can adapt this pesto recipe by using different herbs to change up the flavor. Some herbs that make delicious pesto include basil, cilantro, and parsley. If you'd like to make this recipe more filling, simply add your favorite plant-based or animal-based protein to it.

Per Serving: Calories: 607; Carbohydrates: 104g; Fat: 14g; Saturated Fat: 3g; Sugars: 2g; Cholesterol: 11mg; Protein: 25g; Fiber: 13g; Sodium: 454mg

Spicy Apple and Carrot Salad

SERVES 4 | PREP TIME: 15 MINUTES

30 MINUTES OR LESS • DAIRY-FREE • VEGAN • VEGETARIAN

This is my take on a Thai salad, which hits the perfect balance of sweet, sour, and savory. To make a traditional Thai version, swap the apple for green papaya.

For the dressing

6 tablespoons lime juice

3 tablespoons soy sauce

2 tablespoons honey

2 tablespoons fish sauce (optional)

1 tablespoon lime zest

1 garlic clove, minced

For the salad

2 cups water

2 cups frozen edamame

4 cups carrots, shredded or cut into matchsticks

2 cups Granny Smith apple, cut into matchsticks

2 scallions, finely sliced

½ cup roughly chopped fresh cilantro

½ cup roughly chopped fresh mint or Thai basil

¼ cup roughly chopped peanuts

1 fresh red Thai chile or jalapeño pepper (optional), diced

To make the dressing

1. In a blender, blend the lime juice, soy sauce, honey, fish sauce (if using), lime zest, and garlic until smooth.

To make the salad

2. In a small saucepan, bring the water to a boil. Toss the edamame for 2 to 3 minutes in the boiling water to blanche. Remove the edamame from the saucepan and place it in a large bowl.
3. Add the carrots, apple, and scallions to the bowl. Add the dressing and toss the fruit and vegetables until well coated.
4. Top with the cilantro, mint, peanuts, and chile (if using).

Per Serving: Calories: 249; Carbohydrates: 34g; Fat: 9g; Saturated Fat: 1g; Sugars: 18g; Cholesterol: 0mg; Protein: 14g; Fiber: 9g; Sodium: 660mg

Muffuletta Olive Salad

SERVES 4 | PREP TIME: 15 MINUTES

30 MINUTES OR LESS · DAIRY-FREE · GLUTEN-FREE · NUT-FREE · ONE POT

The muffuletta sandwich is a legendary New Orleans dish created by Sicilian immigrants. Growing up, I recall going to the Italian American deli with my parents to pick up a muffuletta sandwich. To this day, it continues to be one of my favorite things to eat. With this recipe, I wanted to transport you to New Orleans and bring to your table the tangy, bright, umami-rich flavors of the muffuletta. Olives are an excellent source of heart-healthy fats, which help slow down the absorption of carbohydrates into the bloodstream and prevent blood sugar spikes.

1 tablespoon balsamic vinegar

1 teaspoon extra-virgin olive oil

1 garlic clove, minced

2 tablespoons Tuscan Seasoning (page 128), divided

1 celery stalk, finely sliced

2 scallions, finely sliced

½ cup diced green olives

½ cup diced kalamata olives

½ cup diced roasted red bell peppers

2 tablespoons capers, drained

2 cups roasted chicken or canned organic roasted chicken breast, no added salt (optional)

1. In a large bowl, combine the vinegar, oil, garlic, 1 tablespoon of Tuscan seasoning, the celery, scallions, green and kalamata olives, peppers, and capers.

2. In a smaller bowl, season the chicken with the remaining 1 tablespoon of Tuscan seasoning. Place the chicken on top of individual portions of salad or mix it into the entire salad.

3. You can eat this salad immediately or store it in an airtight container in the refrigerator. If you mix the chicken into the salad, it will only keep for up to 3 days in the refrigerator. If you keep the chicken separate, the salad will remain fresh for up to 5 days.

Per Serving: Calories: 63; Carbohydrates: 5g; Fat: 5g; Saturated Fat: 1g; Sugars: 2g; Cholesterol: 0mg; Protein: 1g; Fiber: 2g; Sodium: 359mg

Olive Lentil Arugula Salad

SERVES 4 | PREP TIME: 15 MINUTES | COOK TIME: 25 MINUTES

DAIRY-FREE · GLUTEN-FREE · VEGAN · VEGETARIAN

This salad is the perfect quick and easy lunch, since it provides protein, fiber-rich carbohydrates, healthy fats, and leafy greens. Peppery and spicy, arugula can truly brighten any salad. Arugula is a good source of vitamins C and K, beta-carotene, folate, and calcium, making it a super nutritious leafy green. Diets rich in beta-carotene are linked to healthier blood sugar levels.

For the lentils

2½ cups vegetable broth or water
1 cup French lentils,
    drained and rinsed

¼ medium onion
½ teaspoon turmeric
¼ teaspoon sea salt

For the salad

1 cup kalamata olives, pitted
    or roughly chopped
1 cup pomegranate seeds (optional)
¼ cup walnuts, roasted and
    chopped
¼ cup sunflower or pumpkin
    seeds, roasted or raw

2 tablespoons lemon juice
1 tablespoon balsamic vinegar
2 teaspoons extra-virgin olive oil
1 teaspoon salt
5 cups arugula, washed and dried

To make the lentils

1. In a medium pot, combine the broth, lentils, onion, turmeric, and salt. Cover the pot and bring to a boil over medium heat.
2. Once boiling, reduce the heat to low and simmer uncovered for 20 minutes, until the lentils are tender.
3. Drain the lentils and remove the onion.

To make the salad

4. In a large bowl, combine the lentils, olives, pomegranate seeds (if using), walnuts, sunflower seeds, lemon juice, vinegar, oil, and salt.

5. Add the arugula to the bowl and gently toss all the ingredients until combined.

Technique Tip: Learning to cook dry lentils can help you save money. Cook dry lentils during the weekend and store them in an airtight container in the refrigerator, where they'll remain fresh for up to 5 days. You'll be able to add them to your salads throughout the week as a source of protein.

Per Serving: Calories: 255; Carbohydrates: 24g; Fat: 14g; Saturated Fat: 2g; Sugars: 3g; Cholesterol: 0mg; Protein: 13g; Fiber: 10g; Sodium: 855mg

Roasted Tomato Soup

SERVES 4 | PREP TIME: 10 MINUTES | COOK TIME: 30 MINUTES

DAIRY-FREE · GLUTEN-FREE · NUT-FREE · ONE POT · VEGAN · VEGETARIAN

One of my absolute favorite meals as a child was tomato soup and grilled cheese. I loved dipping my grilled cheese sandwich into my soup bowl. This roasted tomato soup is fiery and flavorful. Made with plant-based ingredients, it is lower in saturated fat than traditional tomato soup, but it remains creamy and smooth. I suggest that you pair it with a salad for the perfect lunch. If you are feeling nostalgic, make yourself a grilled cheese sandwich using whole-wheat bread and cheddar cheese. There's nothing as comforting as dunking a grilled cheese sandwich into your tomato soup.

2½ pounds tomatoes (heirlooms, cherry, vine, or plum), cored and quartered

3 garlic cloves

2 small yellow onions, sliced (about 3 cups)

1 tablespoon extra-virgin olive oil

1 teaspoon salt

½ teaspoon freshly ground black pepper or red pepper flakes

1 tablespoon Tuscan Seasoning (page 128) or Italian seasoning

1 quart vegetable broth

1 bay leaf

2 teaspoons maple syrup (optional)

½ cup chopped fresh basil (optional)

1. Preheat the oven to 425°F. Line a baking sheet with parchment paper.
2. Spread the tomatoes, garlic cloves, and onions on the baking sheet. Drizzle with the oil and season with the salt and pepper, mixing to coat well.
3. Roast the veggies until caramelized, about 20 minutes.
4. Remove the veggies from the oven and place them in a large pot. Add the Tuscan seasoning, vegetable broth, and bay leaf. Stir and bring to a boil over medium-high heat, about 10 minutes. Remove from heat.
5. Remove the bay leaf. Using an immersion blender, a regular blender, or a food processor (see tip), puree the soup until smooth and creamy.

6. Taste the soup. If it's too tart, add the maple syrup.

7. Garnish with the basil (if using).

Technique Tip: If you'd like to turn this soup into a creamy tomato soup, simply stir in ½ cup of coconut cream or Greek yogurt before serving or add a dollop to the individual portions. When blending hot soups, be careful not to splash hot liquid toward your face. If using an immersion blender, pour the soup into a large bowl or pot and tilt the bowl away from your face for blending. If using a stand mixer or blender, do not overfill. Close the lid tightly and place a dry towel over the closed lid while blending.

Per Serving: Calories: 110; Carbohydrates: 18g; Fat: 4g; Saturated Fat: 1g; Sugars: 11g; Cholesterol: 0mg; Protein: 3g; Fiber: 4g; Sodium: 437mg

Lemon Mint Bulgur Salad

SERVES 4 | PREP TIME: 10 MINUTES | COOK TIME: 25 MINUTES

DAIRY-FREE · VEGAN · VEGETARIAN

Bulgur wheat is a protein-rich whole grain that is traditionally used in recipes from diverse countries throughout the Middle East and Africa. Rich in fiber and phytonutrients, bulgur and other whole grains are linked to improved blood glucose levels and gut health. This recipe is simple to put together and will keep in the refrigerator for up to 5 days. It can be eaten warm or cold.

1 cup bulgur

1½ cups vegetable broth or water

½ cup slivered almonds

½ cup capers, drained

¼ cup finely chopped red onion

¼ cup raisins

¼ cup sunflower seeds

¼ cup chopped fresh mint

¼ cup chopped fresh cilantro (optional)

1 tablespoon lemon juice

2 teaspoons extra-virgin olive oil

1. In a medium pot, combine the bulgur and broth. Cover and bring to a boil over medium heat. Once boiling, lower the heat and simmer for 20 minutes or until the bulgur is tender but not mushy.

2. Drain the bulgur if there is excess liquid. Place the drained bulgur in a large bowl and add the almonds, capers, red onion, raisins, sunflower seeds, mint, cilantro (if using), lemon juice, and oil. Stir to combine.

Substitution Tip: If you don't have bulgur handy, you can use quinoa (gluten-free), brown rice (gluten-free), barley, millet (gluten-free), whole-wheat pasta, or other favorite gluten-free whole grains to make this salad. For more gluten-free grains, check out the list on page 27. Add your favorite protein source for added satiety.

Per Serving: Calories: 297; Carbohydrates: 41g; Fat: 13g; Saturated Fat: 1g; Sugars: 8g; Cholesterol: 1mg; Protein: 10g; Fiber: 8g; Sodium: 432mg

Zucchini Basil Soup

SERVES 4 | PREP TIME: 10 MINUTES | COOK TIME: 15 MINUTES

30 MINUTES OR LESS • DAIRY-FREE • GLUTEN-FREE • NUT-FREE • VEGAN • VEGETARIAN

This soup is an excellent option for summer, when zucchini and fresh basil are in season and abundant. Zucchini is a good source of vitamins A and C, manganese, and fiber. Manganese is crucial for healthy bone development, and adding fiber-rich vegetables to your diet promotes gut health and regular bowel movements.

2 teaspoons extra-virgin olive oil
1 medium onion, finely sliced
2 garlic cloves, roughly chopped
1½ pounds zucchini, cut
    into rounds
1½ teaspoons sea salt

1 tablespoon Tuscan Seasoning
    (page 128)
1 (15.5-ounce) can navy beans,
    drained and rinsed
2 cups vegetable low-sodium broth
1 cup fresh basil

1. In a large pot, heat the oil over medium heat. Add the onion, garlic, zucchini, salt, and Tuscan seasoning to the saucepan, reduce the heat to low, and sweat until lightly browned, about 5 minutes.
2. Add the navy beans and vegetable broth and reduce to a simmer. Cover with a lid and simmer until tender, 8 to 10 minutes.
3. Transfer the zucchini mixture to a food processor or blender. Add the basil and salt and puree until smooth.

Substitution Tip: If you don't have fresh basil available, substitute your favorite fresh herb such as mint, cilantro, dill, tarragon, or parsley.

Per Serving: Calories: 127; Carbohydrates: 20g; Fat: 3g; Saturated Fat: 1g; Sugars: 6g; Cholesterol: 0mg; Protein: 6g; Fiber: 7g; Sodium: 887mg

Lemony Oven Roasted Cauliflower and Broccoli with Tahini Dressing

SERVES 4 | PREP TIME: 15 MINUTES | COOK TIME: 15 MINUTES

30 MINUTES OR LESS · DAIRY-FREE · NUT-FREE · VEGAN · VEGETARIAN

This recipe is not your mushy and bland childhood broccoli. Zesty, crunchy, and lusciously creamy, this broccoli and cauliflower recipe will turn you into a super fan of cruciferous veggies! Cruciferous vegetables are excellent sources of fiber, vitamins C and K, and other antioxidants important for immune health, cell repair, and healthy aging. Broccoli is also a good source of plant-based protein and iron.

For the dressing

2 tablespoons tahini

1 tablespoon low-sodium soy sauce

1 tablespoon water

2 teaspoons balsamic vinegar

1 teaspoon maple syrup

For the roasted vegetables

3 tablespoons lemon or lime juice

1 tablespoon balsamic vinegar

2 teaspoons extra-virgin olive oil

1 teaspoon dried basil

1 teaspoon dried oregano

¼ teaspoon salt

1 medium head broccoli, cut into florets

1 medium head cauliflower, cut into florets

To make the dressing

1. In a bowl, whisk together the tahini, soy sauce, water, vinegar, and maple syrup.

To make the roasted vegetables

2. Preheat the oven to 425°F. Line a large baking sheet with parchment paper and set aside.
3. In a large bowl, combine the lemon juice, vinegar, oil, basil, oregano, and salt.

4. Add the broccoli and cauliflower and coat with the mixture. Transfer the broccoli and cauliflower to the lined baking sheet, making sure not to overcrowd it.
5. Bake for 12 minutes or until the vegetables are golden brown. Remove from the oven and set aside to cool.
6. Before serving, toss the vegetables with the dressing. Serve warm, at room temperature, or chilled.

Ingredient Tip: You can also use precut or frozen broccoli and cauliflower. If using frozen broccoli and cauliflower, cook for 5 minutes more. Drizzle this tahini dressing on your favorite salads or roasted vegetables to add creaminess, healthy fat, and protein to your plate.

Per Serving: Calories: 171; Carbohydrates: 23g; Fat: 7g; Saturated Fat: 1g; Sugars: 8g; Cholesterol: 0mg; Protein: 9g; Fiber: 8g; Sodium: 378mg

Warming Ginger Carrot Bisque

SERVES 5 | PREP TIME: 10 MINUTES | COOK TIME: 30 MINUTES

DAIRY-FREE ▪ GLUTEN-FREE ▪ VEGAN ▪ VEGETARIAN

This warming soup is perfect for cold, wintry days and is excellent to drink when you are fighting a cold. This is a great base recipe that can be made with various root vegetables including parsnips, turnips, and yams.

2 teaspoons extra-virgin olive oil

1 medium onion, sliced

1½ teaspoons sea salt

2 pounds carrots, cut into
  ½-inch rounds

¼ cup cashews, raw (optional)

5 cups vegetable broth or water,
  plus more as needed

2 teaspoons grated fresh ginger

1 tablespoon lime juice (½ lime)

2 tablespoons chopped dill,
  for garnish

1. In large stockpot, heat the oil over medium heat. Add the onion and salt. Reduce the heat to low and sweat the onions until they are soft and translucent, about 5 minutes, making sure to avoid browning them.
2. Add the carrots and cashews (if using), cover the pot, and sweat for 5 minutes. Stir to prevent browning.
3. Add the vegetable broth. Raise the heat to medium-high and bring the soup to a boil. Once the soup boils, reduce the heat and simmer with the lid slightly ajar for about 15 minutes, or until the carrots are soft and tender.
4. Transfer the soup to a blender and add the ginger. Blend the soup until it becomes creamy, adding more vegetable broth as needed to achieve your desired texture.
5. Return the soup to the pot and reheat over medium-low. Stir in the lime juice and add more salt to taste.
6. Garnish with the dill and serve.

Per Serving: Calories: 100; Carbohydrates: 20g; Fat: 2g; Saturated Fat: 0g; Sugars: 10g; Cholesterol: 0mg; Protein: 2g; Fiber: 6g; Sodium: 824mg

Three Bean Salad

SERVES 4 | PREP TIME: 15 MINUTES

30 MINUTES OR LESS ▪ **DAIRY-FREE** ▪ **GLUTEN-FREE** ▪ **NUT-FREE** ▪ **ONE POT** ▪ **VEGAN** ▪ **VEGETARIAN**

This hearty bean salad will truly satisfy your hunger and banish any cravings for carbohydrates. You can use this recipe as a side dish, or make it a salad by mixing it with leafy greens. Beans are true prediabetes superfoods and should be a part of your weekly diet. They have a low glycemic index, which means that they don't cause sudden spikes in blood sugar.

1 (15-ounce) can black beans, drained and rinsed

1 (15-ounce) can kidney beans, drained and rinsed

1 (15-ounce) can pinto beans, drained and rinsed

1 (15-ounce) can crushed tomatoes

2 cups green bell peppers, diced

½ cup canned corn, drained and rinsed

¼ cup red onion or scallions, finely chopped

½ cup fresh cilantro or herb of choice, chopped (optional)

2 tablespoons lemon or lime juice

2 teaspoons extra-virgin olive oil

1 teaspoon smoked paprika

1 teaspoon dried oregano

½ teaspoon cumin

½ teaspoon salt

1. In a large bowl, stir together the black beans, kidney beans, pinto beans, tomatoes with their juices, peppers, corn, and onion.
2. In a small bowl, whisk the cilantro (if using), lemon juice, oil, paprika, oregano, cumin, and salt into a vinaigrette.
3. Pour the dressing over the bean mixture, toss well, and add more cilantro, paprika, oregano, cumin, and salt to taste.

Variation Tip: To create a warm bean salad, sauté the onions, tomatoes, and bell peppers in 2 teaspoons of olive oil. Add the remaining ingredients and bring to a simmer.

Per Serving: Calories: 277; Carbohydrates: 44g; Fat: 4g; Saturated Fat: 0g; Sugars: 4g; Cholesterol: 0mg; Protein: 15g; Fiber: 8g; Sodium: 992mg

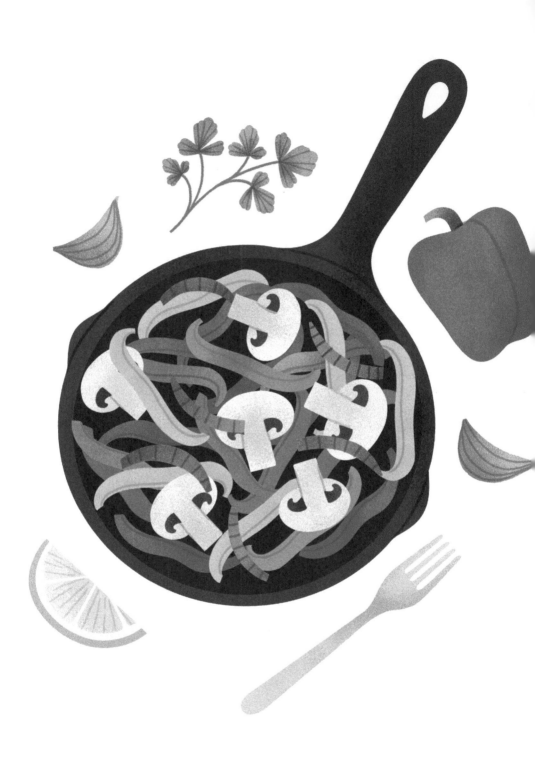

CHAPTER 8

Hearty Mains

Guatemalan-Style Chilaquilas

SERVES 4 | PREP TIME: 20 MINUTES | COOK TIME: 20 MINUTES

DAIRY-FREE · NUT-FREE · VEGETARIAN

Not to be confused with Mexican chilaquiles, this recipe was inspired by Guatemalan chilaquilas, which are a traditional breakfast vegetable and tortilla dish. Eating savory, spicy, fiber-rich meals will help keep your blood sugar balanced throughout the entire day while also keeping you satisfied and energized. This recipe highlights zucchini, which is an excellent source of water, fiber, and antioxidants. The antioxidants in zucchini (including carotenoid) protect against damage from free radicals, which are linked to aging and increased risk of certain cancers. Zucchini consumption is associated with improved insulin sensitivity and healthier blood glucose levels.

For the tortillas

1 tablespoon extra-virgin olive oil

4 whole-wheat or corn tortillas, cut into large squares

For the spicy chipotle salsa

5 tomatillos

2 Roma tomatoes

½ yellow onion (or onion of choice), roughly chopped (about ½ cup)

1 garlic clove

1 teaspoon salt

¼ teaspoon dried chipotle (add more for spicier salsa)

¼ cup water

For the chilaquilas

2 teaspoons butter

4 eggs

2 teaspoons extra-virgin olive oil

4 teaspoons onion (about ¼ medium onion), finely chopped

2 cups zucchini (about 2 medium zucchini), cut into 1-inch dice

4 tablespoons sour cream or vegan sour cream

¼ teaspoon salt

¼ cup queso fresco or Parmesan cheese (optional)

To make the tortillas

1. In a medium skillet, heat the oil over medium heat. When the oil is hot, add the tortillas, stirring occasionally to make sure they do not burn. The tortillas are ready when they look lightly browned and crispy, about 3 minutes.

To make the spicy chipotle salsa

2. Put the tomatillos, tomatoes, onion, garlic, salt, chipotle, and water in a medium saucepan. Cover the saucepan with a lid and bring to a boil over medium heat.
3. Once boiling, remove the pan from the heat and let it cool for a few minutes.
4. Once cool, transfer the contents of the saucepan to a blender, blending until smooth. You may also use an immersion blender, but make sure not to burn yourself while blending.

To make the chilaquilas

5. In a large skillet, melt the butter over medium-high heat. Either scramble or fry the eggs, cooking to your preferred doneness. Remove the eggs from the skillet and set aside.
6. Heat the oil in a large skillet over medium heat. Add the onion and caramelize until lightly browned, about 3 minutes.
7. Add the zucchini to the skillet and cook for 3 to 5 minutes more, until tender but not mushy. Top with sour cream and sprinkle with salt and queso fresco (if using).
8. Top with the cooked eggs, crispy tortillas, and salsa and serve warm.

Substitution Tip: Traditionally in Guatemala, chilaquilas are made with chayote, sometimes called mirliton. Feel free to substitute mirliton for the zucchini if you'd like to try a new vegetable. It's an excellent source of vitamins C and K, folate, and other antioxidants important for health. You can also substitute store-bought salsa for the spicy chipotle salsa if desired.

Per Serving: Calories: 242; Carbohydrates: 19g; Fat: 15g; Saturated Fat: 4g; Sugars: 5g; Cholesterol: 170mg; Protein: 9g; Fiber: 3g; Sodium: 454mg

Veggie Quesadilla

SERVES 4 | PREP TIME: 15 MINUTES | COOK TIME: 20 MINUTES

DAIRY-FREE · GLUTEN-FREE · NUT-FREE · VEGAN · VEGETARIAN

Melty and toasty quesadillas are simple to make and comforting to eat. I fell in love with quesadillas after spending a month in a small port city in Chiapas, Mexico. In Mexico and Latin America, quesadillas are traditionally stuffed with zucchini or fresh zucchini flowers. Quesadillas are the perfect vehicle for adding fiber-rich succulent vegetables and lean protein to your diet.

2 teaspoons extra-virgin olive oil

1 cup baby portobello or white mushrooms, wiped clean and sliced

½ cup thinly sliced onions

½ medium bell pepper, seeded and thinly sliced

1 garlic clove, minced

2 teaspoons Creole Seasoning (page 116)

½ teaspoon ground coriander

½ teaspoon salt

¼ teaspoon ground cumin

½ medium zucchini, cut into matchsticks or half-moons

½ medium yellow squash, cut into matchsticks or half-moons

1 cup cheddar cheese, Monterey Jack cheese, queso fresco, or Homemade Cashew Queso (page 135)

4 large whole-wheat tortillas or 8 small corn tortillas

1 cup of avocado (about ½ medium avocado) (optional)

1. In a large skillet, heat the oil over medium heat. Add the mushrooms and caramelize for 5 to 7 minutes, until the liquid released by the mushrooms evaporates.
2. Add the onion, pepper, garlic, Creole seasoning, coriander, salt, and cumin and cook for 3 minutes.
3. Add the zucchini and yellow squash. Lightly sauté until the veggies are tender, 5 to 7 minutes.
4. Stuff each tortilla with 3 to 4 tablespoons of sautéed veggies and 3 tablespoons of cheddar cheese and fold in half. (If you use cashew cheese, be aware that it will not melt.)

5. Place the tortillas in a skillet over medium-high heat and brown them for 2 to 3 minutes on both sides until they are warm and crunchy and the cheese has melted. Alternatively, you can put the quesadillas in a 350°F toaster oven for about 3 minutes until crispy and melty, or in the microwave for 1 to 2 minutes or until the cheese is melted.
6. Serve with the avocado (if using).

Variation Tip: To make this dish even more filling and protein-rich, add your favorite plant-based or animal protein during step 2, and increase the cooking time as needed to ensure that the protein is thoroughly cooked. Suggestions for protein include ½ cup of tofu per person (see the tofu preparation in the Vegetarian Chipotle Sesame Poke Bowl on page 120) or 3 to 4 ounces of ground meat, turkey, roasted chicken, or steak per person.

Per Serving: Calories: 275; Carbohydrates: 30g; Fat: 13g; Saturated Fat: 6g; Sugars: 4g; Cholesterol: 29mg; Protein: 11g; Fiber: 4g; Sodium: 486mg

Eggplant Chickpea Curry Stew

SERVES 4 | PREP TIME: 15 MINUTES | COOK TIME: 30 MINUTES

DAIRY-FREE ▪ VEGAN ▪ VEGETARIAN

This recipe was inspired by Ayurvedic cooking. Ayurveda is a healing philosophy traditionally practiced in southern India. A few years ago, I spent a month in Kerala learning about Ayurvedic and yoga practices, which included cooking. Through my Ayurvedic studies, I learned about the healing properties of spices. This recipe highlights some of the healing spices treasured in Ayurveda. Turmeric has anti-inflammatory and antioxidant properties. Coriander may help reduce blood sugar levels, cholesterol, and high blood sugar.

For the curry powder

1 tablespoon ground cumin

1 tablespoon ground coriander

1 tablespoon ground ginger

1 tablespoon ground turmeric

1 tablespoon mustard seeds

1 teaspoon ground cardamom

1 teaspoon sweet paprika

For the curry stew

2 teaspoons avocado oil

1 large onion, finely chopped

3 garlic cloves, minced

2 teaspoons finely grated or minced fresh ginger

3 carrots, peeled and cut into bite-size pieces

2 celery stalks, cut into bite-size pieces

½ medium eggplant, cut into large cubes (about 2 cups)

2 (15-ounce) cans chickpeas

1 cup broccoli florets

1 cup cauliflower florets

½ cup coconut milk

2 tablespoons soy sauce (optional)

1 teaspoon honey

1 teaspoon salt

To make the curry powder

1. Mix the cumin, coriander, ginger, turmeric, mustard seeds, cardamom, and paprika in a jar until well combined.

To make the curry stew

2. Heat the oil in a large saucepan or Dutch oven over medium heat. Add the onion, garlic, ginger, and 1 tablespoon of curry powder. Cook until the onions are soft and translucent, stirring occasionally to prevent the garlic from burning, about 5 minutes.
3. Add the carrots, celery, eggplant, and chickpeas to the pan. Cook for about 5 minutes until the carrots and celery start to become tender.
4. Add the broccoli and cauliflower and cook for 5 minutes more, with the lid on.
5. Reduce the heat to low, and then pour the coconut milk, soy sauce (if using), honey, and salt into the pan and stir until all the vegetables and chickpeas are well coated.
6. Cover the pan with a lid and cook for 10 minutes more, or until all the vegetables are tender, making sure that the coconut milk doesn't burn. If the liquid evaporates, add water to the pot.
7. Serve hot.

Variation Tip: You can add chicken or tofu to this recipe. Simply add the chicken after step 1 and sauté in the oil for about 8 minutes until browned. If adding tofu, add it in step 4. Continue to follow the recipe as written. Serve with your favorite cooked whole grain.

Per Serving: Calories: 328; Carbohydrates: 46g; Fat: 13g; Saturated Fat: 7g; Sugars: 14g; Cholesterol: 0mg; Protein: 12g; Fiber: 14g; Sodium: 886mg

New Orleans–Style Red Beans

SERVES 4 | PREP TIME: 15 MINUTES | COOK TIME: 15 MINUTES

30 MINUTES OR LESS • DAIRY-FREE • NUT-FREE • VEGAN • VEGETARIAN

This recipe is inspired by a New Orleans classic that is a staple in my hometown. Red beans are traditionally made with sausage; however, in this interpretation, we add fiber and flavor by using meaty, decadent mushrooms. Serve this recipe on its own or with a mindful side portion of your favorite rice.

For the Creole seasoning

2 teaspoons smoked paprika

1 teaspoon salt

1 teaspoon dried oregano

½ teaspoon dried thyme

¼ teaspoon garlic powder

¼ teaspoon celery salt

¼ teaspoon red pepper flakes

For the red beans

1 tablespoon extra-virgin olive oil

12 button or cremini mushrooms, thinly sliced or roughly chopped

2 bay leaves

½ cup Italian sausage, ground beef, turkey, chicken, or meat substitute like Upton's Naturals Seitan Chorizo (optional)

1 cup diced onion

2 celery stalks, finely sliced

2 red bell peppers, seeded and cut in ½-inch dice

4 garlic cloves, minced

½ teaspoon salt

2 (15-ounce) cans red kidney beans, drained and rinsed

3 cups vegetable broth

To make the Creole seasoning

1. Mix the paprika, salt, oregano, thyme, garlic powder, celery salt, and red pepper flakes in a jar until well combined.

To make the red beans

2. Heat the oil in a large pot over medium-high heat.
3. Once the oil is hot, add the mushrooms, bay leaves, and sausage (if using). Sauté until the mushrooms begin to soften and smell aromatic, about 5 minutes.
4. Add the onion, celery, bell peppers, garlic, and salt and sauté until the vegetables are tender. Sprinkle with the Creole seasoning.
5. Add the red kidney beans to the pot, stir, and sauté for about 2 minutes to bloom the spices and allow the beans to mix with the vegetables.
6. Add the vegetable broth and let it come to a simmer, 5 to 7 minutes.

Serving Tip: Serve with ½ cup of cooked rice or your favorite whole grain, a side salad, or roasted vegetables.

Per Serving: Calories: 300; Carbohydrates: 40g; Fat: 8g; Saturated Fat: 2g; Sugars: 5g; Cholesterol: 10mg; Protein: 18g; Fiber: 15g; Sodium: 512mg

Ginger Sesame Roasted Salmon

SERVES 4 | PREP TIME: 10 MINUTES, PLUS 15 MINUTES OR MORE TO MARINATE | COOK TIME: 15 MINUTES

DAIRY-FREE · NUT-FREE

My preferred animal protein is fish due to its content of omega-3s, which are linked to lower blood pressure and inflammation. When I purchase salmon (or any other seafood), I prioritize freshness and sustainability. If you'd like to check for ethically and sustainably fished or farmed salmon, please visit SeafoodWatch.org. This website was created by the Monterey Bay Aquarium, a leading research organization on sustainability and seafood.

For the ginger sesame marinade

¼ cup white miso (or miso of choice)

¼ cup warm water

2 tablespoons mirin (Japanese cooking wine), dry sherry, or water

2 tablespoons soy sauce

1 tablespoon lime juice

2 teaspoons sesame oil

2 teaspoons grated fresh ginger

1 garlic clove, minced

1 teaspoon extra-virgin olive oil

1 teaspoon honey

½ teaspoon freshly ground black pepper

For the salmon

1 pound salmon, divided into 4 (4-ounce) portions (skin removed or on)

¼ teaspoon salt

1 teaspoon avocado oil or extra-virgin olive oil

To make the ginger sesame marinade

1. In a small bowl, dissolve the miso in the warm water.
2. In a medium bowl, combine the dissolved miso, mirin, soy sauce, lime juice, sesame oil, ginger, garlic, olive oil, honey, and pepper. Whisk together until the ingredients are well combined.

To make the salmon

3. Preheat the oven to 425°F.
4. Place the salmon fillets in a shallow casserole dish, sprinkle them with the salt, and pour the marinade over them. Let the salmon marinate for at least 15 minutes. (The longer the fillets marinate, the more flavorful they'll be. If you are marinating for longer than 15 minutes, store the salmon in the refrigerator.)
5. Lightly oil a baking sheet or oven-safe casserole dish. Arrange the fillets, skin-side down, on the baking sheet and bake for about 12 minutes.

Variation Tip: You can use this marinade to prepare tuna belly and any other type of fish. It also makes an excellent marinade for extra-firm tofu. If you don't want to roast the salmon, you can pan-fry it on the stovetop using a nonstick skillet or grill it for 4 to 5 minutes on each side.

Serving Tip: Serve the salmon with sautéed greens or a kale salad and a cup of your favorite cooked whole grains.

Per Serving: Calories: 190; Carbohydrates: 3g; Fat: 9g; Saturated Fat: 1g; Sugars: 2g; Cholesterol: 63mg; Protein: 23g; Fiber: 0g; Sodium: 473mg

Vegetarian Chipotle Sesame Poke Bowl

SERVES 4 | PREP TIME: 15 MINUTES | COOK TIME: 35 MINUTES

DAIRY-FREE · VEGAN · VEGETARIAN

Poke bowls are a refreshing, light, sweet, and sour dish traditional to Hawaii. This poke bowl is packed with vitamins and fiber-rich vegetables and fruit that will help keep you full. In addition to vegetables, this recipe also features tofu, an excellent source of protein. To achieve a crispier tofu, it is important to properly dry and press the tofu. Wrap the tofu in paper towels or clean kitchen towels, and then place the tofu on a cutting board and put a heavy object on top (like a skillet or bag of rice) to squeeze out any excess water. You can also purchase a tofu presser. The longer you let your tofu press, the crispier your tofu will be when you cook it.

For the chipotle sesame marinade

1½ cups canned crushed tomatoes or tomato puree

¼ cup apple juice

3 garlic cloves, minced

1 tablespoon sesame oil

1 tablespoon maple syrup

1 tablespoon apple cider vinegar

2 teaspoons Dijon mustard (or mustard of choice)

1 teaspoon ground cumin

1 teaspoon ground coriander

¾ teaspoon salt

¼ teaspoon chipotle chili powder or dried crushed chipotle peppers

¼ teaspoon smoked paprika

For the poke bowl

2 pounds extra-firm tofu, drained and pressed

2 teaspoons extra-virgin olive oil

2 cups salad greens

1 cup cooked whole grain (white or brown rice, quinoa, millet, barley)

½ cup avocado, pitted and diced

¼ cup mango, cut in 1-inch dice (optional)

1 tablespoon pickled ginger (optional)

½ cup frozen edamame, blanched (optional)

To make the chipotle sesame marinade

1. In a blender, blend the tomatoes, apple juice, garlic, sesame oil, maple syrup, vinegar, mustard, cumin, coriander, salt, chili powder, and paprika until smooth. Set aside. The marinade may be stored in a jar or sealed container in the refrigerator for up to 1 week or in the freezer for up to 3 months.

To make the poke bowl

2. Cut the tofu into 1-inch pieces and place in a bowl. Drizzle with the oil.
3. In a large skillet over medium heat, sear the tofu for 4 to 5 minutes on each side. You may need to sear the tofu in two batches if your skillet is not large enough.
4. Add 2 cups of marinade to the skillet. Simmer for about 15 minutes, until the sauce is warm and bubbling.
5. Assemble the poke bowls by layering salad greens, whole grains, tofu, avocado, mango (if using), pickled ginger (if using), and edamame (if using). Enjoy!

Variation Tip: Alternatively, use the Ginger Sesame Marinade (page 118) to season the tofu. If you have leftover salmon, tuna salad, or ceviche, you can substitute fish for tofu in this recipe.

Per Serving: Calories: 431; Carbohydrates: 37g; Fat: 23g; Saturated Fat: 2g; Sugars: 16g; Cholesterol: 0mg; Protein: 27g; Fiber: 6g; Sodium: 524mg

Tofu Stir-Fry

SERVES 4 | PREP TIME: 15 MINUTES | COOK TIME: 25 MINUTES

DAIRY-FREE · GLUTEN-FREE · NUT-FREE · ONE POT · VEGAN · VEGETARIAN

Once you know how to make a stir-fry, you can use it as your go-to meal when you are pressed for time. You can add any protein or vegetable to a stir-fry, so if you don't have one of the ingredients on hand, just toss in what you do have. The key is to add the firmer vegetables first, followed by the quicker-cooking vegetables.

3 teaspoons avocado or canola oil, divided

1 (14-ounce) block extra-firm tofu, drained and pressed, cut in 1-inch dice

2 cups carrots, shredded or cut into bite-size pieces

1 cup broccoli florets

1 cup sliced red bell pepper

1 cup Brussels sprouts, halved (optional)

½ cup red cabbage, finely shredded (optional)

1 cup frozen edamame

4 garlic cloves, minced

2 teaspoons minced or grated fresh ginger

3 tablespoons soy sauce

1 teaspoon sesame oil

3 teaspoons sesame seeds (optional)

4 scallions, thinly sliced

1. In a large skillet or wok over high heat, heat 2 teaspoons of avocado oil until hot and shimmering. Add the tofu to the skillet and sear until golden brown on all sides, about 2 minutes per side. Remove the tofu from the skillet.

2. Heat the remaining 1 teaspoon of avocado oil over high heat.

3. Add the carrots, broccoli, pepper, and Brussels sprouts (if using) to the skillet and stir-fry over medium-high heat until the vegetables soften and brown slightly, about 5 minutes.

4. Add the cabbage (if using) and edamame and continue to stir-fry until the vegetables are tender and golden brown, 3 to 5 minutes.

5. Lower the heat to medium and add the garlic, ginger, soy sauce, sesame oil, and sesame seeds (if using). Cook for 2 minutes, making sure to stir constantly to prevent the garlic and sesame seeds from burning. Remove from heat.
6. Top with the scallions.

Variation Tip: If you want to add more protein to this dish or replace the tofu, you can use your favorite animal protein. If you are cooking an animal protein, add it during step 1, making sure it is thoroughly cooked before moving on to the next steps. You can also add scrambled eggs to this recipe, but prepare them in a separate skillet and add them to your stir-fry just before serving.

Serving Tip: Serve with 1 cup of your favorite rice, noodles, or whole grains.

Per Serving: Calories: 231; Carbohydrates: 17g; Fat: 13g; Saturated Fat: 1g; Sugars: 6g; Cholesterol: 0mg; Protein: 17g; Fiber: 6g; Sodium: 719mg

Vegetarian (or Not) Fajitas

SERVES 4 | PREP TIME: 15 MINUTES | COOK TIME: 15 MINUTES

30 MINUTES OR LESS • DAIRY-FREE • NUT-FREE • VEGAN • VEGETARIAN

Filled with fiber-rich vegetables, this Tex Mex–inspired fajita recipe is fragrant, aromatic, and perfectly spiced. It will also allow you to enjoy tortillas without worrying about raising your blood sugar. The basic recipe makes a vegetarian version, but a variety of protein choices can easily be added to make a heartier dish.

½ teaspoon extra-virgin olive oil

3 cups mushrooms, thinly sliced

2 cups thinly sliced white or red onions

1½ cups finely chopped red, orange, yellow, or green bell pepper

2 garlic cloves, finely minced

1 teaspoon smoked paprika

1 teaspoon dried oregano

½ teaspoon ground coriander

½ teaspoon salt

¼ teaspoon ground cumin

4 large whole-wheat or corn tortillas

Optional toppings

Cheese

Sour cream

Guacamole

Refried beans

Pico de gallo or salsa

Lime wedges

Fresh cilantro

Optional protein

Chicken

Tofu

Seitan

Ground beef or steak

1. In a large skillet, heat the oil over medium-high heat.
2. Add the mushrooms and cook until they begin to soften, 5 to 7 minutes, making sure to stir occasionally.
3. Add the onion, pepper, garlic, paprika, oregano, coriander, salt, and cumin. Cook until the vegetables are tender but not mushy, about 7 minutes.

4. Warm the tortillas in the microwave for 45 seconds or heat them in a skillet.

5. Place the tortillas on a plate and evenly spoon the fajita filling into each tortilla. Top as desired.

Ingredient Tip: If using a protein option, add it during step 3 and cook to the desired doneness, making sure to fully cook the protein. To prevent the tortillas from drying out when heated in the microwave, wrap them in a damp paper towel or dish towel.

Variation Tip: If you don't have time to measure out the dry spices, you can use Creole Seasoning (page 116) to spice up the fajitas.

Per Serving: Calories: 141; Carbohydrates: 30g; Fat: 2g; Saturated Fat: 0g; Sugars: 13g; Cholesterol: 0mg; Protein: 4g; Fiber: 3g; Sodium: 301mg

Creole-Style Shrimp Étouffée

SERVES 4 | PREP TIME: 10 MINUTES | COOK TIME: 30 MINUTES

DAIRY-FREE · GLUTEN-FREE · ONE POT

Shrimp étouffée is the quintessential New Orleans dish, highlighting Creole cooking techniques and traditional spice blends. This dish provides all the elements you need to achieve healthy blood sugar levels including protein, fiber, and healthy fats.

1 tablespoon extra-virgin olive oil

1 large onion, finely chopped

3 celery stalks, minced

1 small green bell pepper, seeded and finely chopped

1½ teaspoons sea salt

4 garlic cloves, minced

½ teaspoon cayenne pepper

¼ teaspoon red pepper flakes

2 bay leaves

1 (28-ounce) can crushed tomatoes

4½ teaspoons honey or maple syrup

3 pounds medium shrimp (21 to 25 per pound), peeled and deveined

3 scallions, finely sliced

1. In a medium Dutch oven, heat the oil over medium heat.
2. Reduce the heat to low and add the onion, celery, bell pepper, salt, garlic, cayenne pepper, red pepper flakes, and bay leaves. Sweat until the onions are translucent and vegetables are tender and aromatic, about 5 minutes.
3. Raise the heat to medium-high and add the crushed tomatoes. Sauté until the tomatoes caramelize, about 10 minutes.
4. Lower the heat and add the honey. Simmer on low until the sauce thickens, about 5 minutes.
5. Add the shrimp and cook for 5 to 7 minutes more. Add more salt, cayenne pepper, and red pepper flakes to taste and serve topped with the scallions.

Variation Tip: For a vegetarian version, substitute chickpeas or tofu for the shrimp and follow the instructions as listed.

Per Serving: Calories: 404; Carbohydrates: 19g; Fat: 6g; Saturated Fat: 1g; Sugars: 13g; Cholesterol: 548mg; Protein: 71g; Fiber: 6g; Sodium: 1535mg

Meatball Pita Sandwich

SERVES 4 | PREP TIME: 15 MINUTES | COOK TIME: 20 MINUTES

DAIRY-FREE • **NUT-FREE**

In New York City, there are so many Israeli, Syrian, and Lebanese food carts and small food joints that make the most delicious pita sandwiches. It's my love for this zesty street food that inspired this recipe, which is packed with fiber and protein in every bite.

Extra-virgin olive oil, for greasing
1 cup roughly chopped baby portobello mushrooms
1 cup roughly chopped white onion
1 (15-ounce) can black beans, drained and rinsed
1 tablespoon tomato paste
2 teaspoons smoked paprika

2 teaspoons dried oregano
2 teaspoons dried basil
2 teaspoons salt
1 (20-ounce) package lean ground turkey
1 cup bread crumbs
4 whole-wheat pitas, warmed

1. Preheat the oven to 375°F and line a 9-inch baking sheet with parchment paper. Lightly grease the parchment paper with oil.
2. In a food processor, pulse the mushrooms, onion, and black beans until well combined.
3. To the food processor, add the tomato paste, paprika, oregano, basil, and salt. Pulse until mixed.
4. Move the mixture from the food processor to a large bowl. Add the turkey and bread crumbs to the bowl and use your hands to mix.
5. Roll the mixture into 1-inch meatballs. Place the meatballs about 1 inch apart on the prepared baking sheet.
6. Bake the meatballs for 20 minutes, rotating them halfway through.
7. Serve in the whole-wheat pitas.

Substitution Tip: For plant-based meatballs, you can use a 14-ounce block of extra-firm tofu, dried and pressed. Add it to the food processor in step 3 and blend until well incorporated, then go straight to step 5.

Per Serving: Calories: 527; Carbohydrates: 52g; Fat: 19g; Saturated Fat: 4g; Sugars: 3g; Cholesterol: 105mg; Protein: 40g; Fiber: 11g; Sodium: 996mg

Mediterranean-Style Vegetable Cassoulet

SERVES 4 | PREP TIME: 15 MINUTES | COOK TIME: 15 MINUTES

30 MINUTES OR LESS · DAIRY-FREE · GLUTEN-FREE · NUT-FREE · ONE POT · VEGAN · VEGETARIAN

This recipe was inspired by the time I spent in Florence, Italy, learning about food-to-table traditions and Italian cooking. This soup is as comforting as a hug. It is fiber-rich, which promotes balanced blood sugar levels and will help you feel satisfied.

For the Tuscan seasoning

4 tablespoons dried basil

2 tablespoons dried oregano

¼ teaspoon dried thyme

¼ teaspoon red pepper flakes (use ½ teaspoon for a spicier blend)

¼ teaspoon dried rosemary

For the vegetable cassoulet

1 tablespoon extra-virgin olive oil

1 cup diced onion or leek

1 cup sliced carrot

1 celery stalk, cut into bite-size pieces

1 cup diced red bell pepper

3 tablespoons tomato paste

3 garlic cloves, minced

1 teaspoon salt

1 cup chopped green beans

1 (15.5-ounce) can kidney beans, drained and rinsed

6 cups vegetable broth or water

To make the Tuscan seasoning

1. In a bowl or mason jar, combine the basil, oregano, thyme, red pepper flakes, and rosemary and stir until well blended. Store in an airtight container.

To make the vegetable cassoulet

2. In a large stockpot, heat the oil over medium-high heat.
3. Add the onion, carrot, celery, and bell pepper and cook until the vegetables are tender and aromatic, 5 to 6 minutes. Make sure to stir occasionally.

4. Add 1 tablespoon of Tuscan seasoning, the tomato paste, garlic, and salt and sauté until aromatic and well mixed with the vegetables, 3 to 4 minutes.
5. Add the green beans, kidney beans, and vegetable broth. Let simmer for about 5 minutes or until the vegetables are tender but not mushy.

Ingredient Tip: Use this recipe as your go-to comfort soup. Add chicken, Italian sausage, plant-based sausage, seitan, or tempeh to make the soup richer. You can add your protein of choice in step 2 along with the onion.

Per Serving: Calories: 169; Carbohydrates: 27g; Fat: 8g; Saturated Fat: 1g; Sugars: 6g; Cholesterol: 0mg; Protein: 8g; Fiber: 8g; Sodium: 624mg

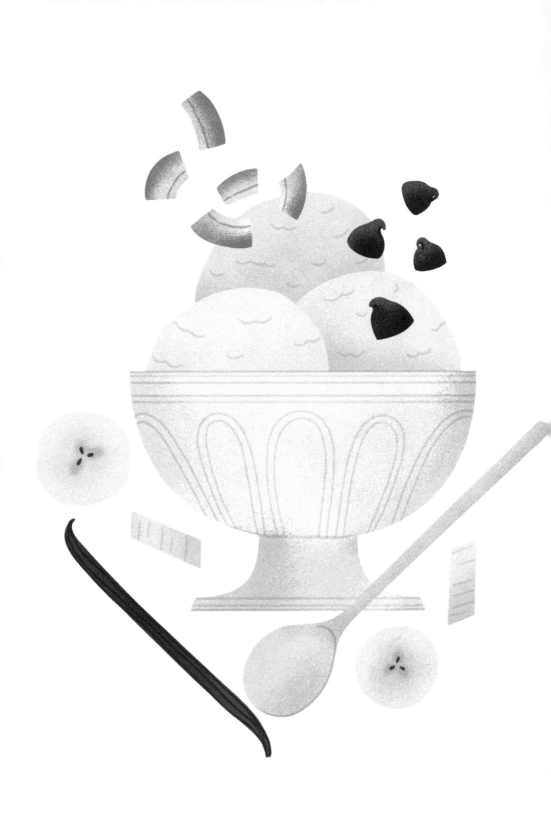

CHAPTER 9

Snacks, Sides, and Sweets

Zesty Guacamole

MAKES 2 CUPS | PREP TIME: 10 MINUTES

30 MINUTES OR LESS · DAIRY-FREE · GLUTEN-FREE · NUT-FREE · ONE POT · VEGAN · VEGETARIAN

One of my favorite foods growing up was guacamole. This is my mom's delicious and tangy recipe, inspired by her childhood in Guatemala. Use this as a substitute for mayonnaise on sandwiches, a creamy addition to salads, or a dip for veggies. It's also perfect to use on avocado toast for a delightful breakfast or healthy snack.

2 ripe medium avocados, halved and pitted

½ cup fresh cilantro, roughly chopped

3 tablespoons lime juice (2 limes)

2 tablespoons fresh jalapeño pepper, minced

1 tablespoon red onion (or onion of choice), finely chopped

1 teaspoon dried Mexican oregano or Italian oregano

¼ teaspoon salt

1. Using a spoon, scoop out the avocado flesh and place it in a medium mixing bowl.
2. Using a fork, mash the avocado to the consistency you desire.
3. Add the cilantro, lime juice, jalapeño pepper, onion, oregano, and salt and mix until well incorporated.

Per Serving (½ cup): Calories: 189; Carbohydrates: 14g; Fat: 15g; Saturated Fat: 3g; Sugars: 4g; Cholesterol: 0mg; Protein: 4g; Fiber: 9g; Sodium: 150mg

Pico de Gallo

MAKES 1¼ CUPS | PREP TIME: 10 MINUTES

30 MINUTES OR LESS ▪ **DAIRY-FREE** ▪ **GLUTEN-FREE** ▪ **NUT-FREE** ▪
ONE POT ▪ **VEGAN** ▪ **VEGETARIAN**

Beloved in Latin America and Southwest United States, pico de gallo will spice up any dish. Although the terms *pico de gallo* and *salsa* are often used interchangeably, you may be interested to learn that they are prepared differently. Salsa is usually made using cooked ingredients like dried peppers and tomatillos. The ingredients used in salsa vary by regions. Pico de gallo is made using fresh ingredients that typically include tomatoes, cilantro, onions, limes, and spicy peppers. Tomatoes have a low glycemic index, meaning that they do not raise blood sugar levels. A diet rich in tomatoes is protective against cancer and linked to improved heart health.

2 medium tomatoes, diced
¼ medium onion, chopped
½ cup cilantro, roughly chopped

2 tablespoons lime juice
½ teaspoon salt

In a medium bowl, mix the tomatoes, onion, cilantro, lime juice, and salt. Serve immediately or store in the refrigerator in an airtight container. Pico de gallo will keep fresh for up to 5 days in the refrigerator.

Substitution Tip: If you don't like cilantro, you can substitute flat-leaf parsley. For a quicker prep, toss the ingredients together in a food processor and pulse to the desired consistency.

Per Serving (¼ cup): Calories: 13; Carbohydrates: 3g; Fat: 0g; Saturated Fat: 0g; Sugars: 2g; Cholesterol: 0mg; Protein: 1g; Fiber: 1g; Sodium: 236mg

Heart-Healthy Refried Black Beans

SERVES 4 | PREP TIME: 5 MINUTES | COOK TIME: 10 MINUTES

30 MINUTES OR LESS · DAIRY-FREE · GLUTEN-FREE · NUT-FREE · ONE POT · VEGAN · VEGETARIAN

The word *fried* may automatically make you think that refried beans are unhealthy. You'll be pleasantly surprised to learn that although some authentic refried bean recipes use lard, refried beans in Latin America are traditionally prepared using safflower, canola, vegetable or—my favorite heart-healthy oil—olive oil. Beans are an excellent source of fiber and protein, making them the perfect food to promote healthy blood sugar levels. Use refried beans as a filling or side dish for enchiladas or chilaquiles, or on top of salads.

2 teaspoons extra-virgin olive oil
¼ cup finely diced onion
¼ cup diced green bell pepper

1 (15-ounce) can black beans, drained and rinsed
½ teaspoon salt
½ teaspoon dried oregano

1. In a large skillet, heat the oil over medium heat.
2. Once the oil is hot, add the onion and pepper and sauté for 3 to 5 minutes, until the onion is translucent and aromatic and the pepper is tender.
3. Add the black beans, salt, and oregano. Simmer for 7 minutes to allow the flavors to combine.

Technique Tip: Use this recipe to kick up the flavor of your favorite types of beans, lentils, or grains. This simple recipe will make any legume or grain richly savory and delightfully filled with umami.

Per Serving: Calories: 105; Carbohydrates: 16g; Fat: 3g; Saturated Fat: 0g; Sugars: 1g; Cholesterol: 0mg; Protein: 6g; Fiber: 6g; Sodium: 292mg

Homemade Cashew Queso

MAKES 2 CUPS | PREP TIME: 10 MINUTES

**30 MINUTES OR LESS · DAIRY-FREE · GLUTEN-FREE · ONE POT ·
VEGAN · VEGETARIAN**

Making homemade, plant-based cheese is a creative way to add more vegetables, healthy fats, and protein to your diet while having fun in the kitchen. If you've never eaten or prepared vegan cheese, you may be wondering what this queso will taste like. This plant-based cheese truly tastes like your favorite cheese puff or cheesy chips. Miso paste, an excellent source of probiotics needed for optimal digestion, is the secret ingredient that makes this queso ooze tangy and nutty flavors. I love to drizzle this velvety queso on quesadillas, fajitas, tacos, popcorn, nachos, and salads.

2 cups raw cashews

1 garlic clove

¾ cup boiling water

½ cup pumpkin puree

3 tablespoons white miso

2 teaspoons tomato puree

½ teaspoon lime or lemon juice

1. Combine the cashews, garlic, water, pumpkin puree, miso, tomato puree, and lime juice in a blender or food processor until creamy.
2. Transfer to an airtight storage container and refrigerate to cool and solidify. The cheese will stay fresh for up to 5 days in the refrigerator.

Substitution Tip: If you are allergic to cashews, you can substitute pumpkin or sunflower seeds. The cheese will be creamier if you use a blender or food processor. However, if you don't have either and your cheese is not blending smoothly, you can soak the cashews or seeds overnight to soften them, or you can do a quick soak. To do a quick soak, in a medium bowl, combine 3 cups of boiling water and the cashews or seeds. Cover with a lid and let soak for 10 to 15 minutes. You can also soak cashews or seeds overnight for the creamiest textures.

Per Serving (¼ cup): Calories: 226; Carbohydrates: 15g; Fat: 17g; Saturated Fat: 3g; Sugars: 3g; Cholesterol: 0mg; Protein: 8g; Fiber: 2g; Sodium: 243mg

Balsamic-Glazed Mushrooms and Chickpeas

SERVES 4 | PREP TIME: 10 MINUTES | COOK TIME: 12 MINUTES

30 MINUTES OR LESS · DAIRY-FREE · GLUTEN-FREE · NUT-FREE · ONE POT · VEGAN · VEGETARIAN

I make this recipe on a weekly basis and keep a batch of it in my refrigerator. Cooking mushrooms using this technique will lead to meaty, tender, smoky mushrooms that make the perfect side dish, filling for a taco, or topping for a salad. Mushrooms are rich in beta-glucan, a type a soluble fiber that is linked to improved cholesterol and blood glucose levels.

2 teaspoons extra-virgin olive oil

1 (8-ounce) package baby portobello mushrooms, wiped clean and sliced

1 cup finely sliced onions

1 (15-ounce) can chickpeas, drained and rinsed

3 garlic cloves, minced

2 tablespoons mirin or sherry (optional)

1 tablespoon balsamic vinegar

2 teaspoons smoked paprika

¾ teaspoon salt

1. In a large skillet, heat the oil over medium heat. Once the oil is hot, add the sliced mushrooms and cook uncovered for 5 to 7 minutes until the liquid released by the mushrooms evaporates.

2. Add the onions, chickpeas, garlic, mirin (if using), vinegar, paprika, and salt and continue to cook for 5 minutes more, or until the onions are caramelized, stirring occasionally to prevent the garlic from burning. Serve as a side dish, salad topping, or avocado toast topping.

Substitution Tip: This recipe is versatile, so you can use any type of mushroom—portobello, shiitake, oyster, porcini, chanterelle—to prepare it. Just make sure your mushrooms are clean! I recommend using a wet paper towel to gently wipe the mushrooms and remove any excess dirt.

Per Serving: Calories: 133; Carbohydrates: 20g; Fat: 4g; Saturated Fat: 0g; Sugars: 6g; Cholesterol: 0mg; Protein: 6g; Fiber: 5g; Sodium: 465mg

Honeydew Melon and Almond Gazpacho

SERVES 4 | PREP TIME: 15 MINUTES

30 MINUTES OR LESS · DAIRY-FREE · GLUTEN-FREE · VEGAN · VEGETARIAN

Gazpacho is a tangy-sweet cold soup traditional to Spain. This refreshing dish is perfect to serve during a barbecue or picnic. Since it is eaten cold and there is no cooking required, it is very quick and easy to make. Honeydew melon is an excellent source of vitamin C, which is crucial to immune, skin, nail, and hair health. Including foods rich in vitamin C may be protective against diabetes, since they may help keep blood sugar levels balanced.

6 cups fresh baby spinach

3 cups cubed honeydew melon

2 cups cubed cucumber

1 cup fresh basil

½ cup slivered almonds

1 garlic clove (optional)

1 shallot

1½ teaspoons salt

3 tablespoons lime juice

1 tablespoon sherry or apple cider vinegar

1 teaspoon extra-virgin olive oil

In a blender, blend the spinach, honeydew, cucumber, basil, almonds, garlic (if using), shallot, salt, lime juice, sherry, and olive oil until smooth. Add more salt and lime juice to taste.

Ingredient Tip: If you're allergic to almonds, you may omit them. You can use your favorite fresh herbs to change the taste profile. The gazpacho should remain fresh in the refrigerator for 3 to 4 days.

Per Serving: Calories: 186; Carbohydrates: 21g; Fat: 11g; Saturated Fat: 1g; Sugars: 13g; Cholesterol: 0mg; Protein: 6g; Fiber: 5g; Sodium: 62mg

Hearts of Palm Ceviche

SERVES 4 | PREP TIME: 20 MINUTES

30 MINUTES OR LESS · DAIRY-FREE · NUT-FREE · VEGAN · VEGETARIAN

Ceviche is a beloved Latin American dish traditionally prepared by curing raw fish in citrus juice. This is my plant-based version of ceviche, which also allows you to incorporate shrimp or tuna. Since the shrimp or tuna you're using will already be cooked, you don't need to worry about purchasing fresh fish that is specially designed to cure in citrus juice. This recipe also uses nori, a seaweed traditional in Japanese cuisine. Nori is a good source of vitamins, minerals, fiber, and antioxidants. Recent studies suggest that seaweed may aid in improving blood sugar control.

For the pickled red onions

3 tablespoons apple cider vinegar

1 tablespoon maple syrup

¼ teaspoon salt

¼ teaspoon freshly ground black pepper

½ cup diced red onion

For the ceviche

2 (14-ounce) cans hearts of palm, drained, divided

2 tablespoons dried nori (seaweed) (optional)

½ cup chopped fresh cilantro (or fresh herb of choice)

½ jalapeño pepper, diced

1 (5-ounce) can tuna, drained (optional)

2 cups jumbo shrimp, deveined and boiled (optional)

2 tablespoons lime juice

½ teaspoon salt

To make the pickled red onions

1. In a large bowl, mix the apple cider vinegar, maple syrup, salt, and black pepper.
2. Add the onions and allow them to marinate while you prepare the rest of the ceviche.
3. Drain and discard the pickling liquid, saving the onions for the ceviche.

To make the ceviche

4. Cut 1 can of the hearts of palm into rings to resemble calamari, and then chop the remaining 1 can of hearts of palm into ½-inch dice.
5. Using kitchen scissors, cut the nori (if using) into thin strips.
6. Mix the hearts of palm, cilantro, jalapeño pepper, pickled onions, tuna (if using), shrimp (if using), and nori (if using). Dress with the lime juice and salt.

Per Serving: Calories: 250; Carbohydrates: 56g; Fat: 0g; Saturated Fat: 0g; Sugars: 38g; Cholesterol: 0mg; Protein: 6g; Fiber: 3g; Sodium: 466mg

Raspberry Crumble Bars

MAKES ABOUT 5 BARS | PREP TIME: 15 MINUTES
COOK TIME: 35 MINUTES

DAIRY-FREE · NUT-FREE · VEGAN · VEGETARIAN

These delicious, tender crumble bars will truly satisfy your sweet tooth. Made with real raspberries and lightly sweetened, this is a dessert that is perfect to share with friends and family. In this recipe, I use chia seeds instead of cornstarch to thicken the raspberry marmalade. Chia seeds are native to Central America and Mexico. One of the most nutritious seeds, chia seeds are a great source of protein, fiber, antioxidants, and healthy fats.

For the raspberry chia seed marmalade

2 cups fresh or frozen raspberries
3 tablespoons maple syrup
2 tablespoons chia seeds

1 teaspoon vanilla extract
⅛ teaspoon salt

For the bars

¼ cup coconut oil
⅓ cup dark brown sugar
⅓ cup white sugar, coconut sugar,
   or raw sugar
1½ cups almond flour
1 cup whole-wheat pastry flour,
   all-purpose flour, or gluten-
   free flour

1 teaspoon salt
½ teaspoon ground cinnamon
¼ teaspoon ground nutmeg
2 tablespoons milk (dairy
   or plant-based)
1 tablespoon orange juice
1 teaspoon orange zest

To make the raspberry chia seed marmalade

1. In a small saucepan over medium heat, combine the raspberries, maple syrup, chia seeds, vanilla, and salt and bring to a boil.
2. Reduce the heat and allow to simmer, uncovered, for about 7 minutes.
3. Remove from heat and allow to cool while you prepare the crumble bars.

4. Preheat the oven to 375°F and line a loaf pan with parchment paper.
5. In a medium mixing bowl, beat the coconut oil and brown and white sugars until fluffy and well combined, about 2 minutes, making sure not to overmix.
6. In a separate bowl, combine the almond flour, pastry flour, salt, cinnamon, and nutmeg and gently whisk together.
7. Add the dry ingredient mixture, milk, orange juice, and orange zest to the coconut sugar mixture. Mix until a crumbly dough forms that does not completely hold together.
8. Press about three-quarters of the dough into the bottom of the loaf pan.
9. Pour about 1 cup of raspberry marmalade into the crust and then crumble the remaining crust mixture on top of the filling.
10. Bake for 30 to 35 minutes or until the crust is golden.
11. Remove the pan from the oven and set aside on a cooling rack. Once cool, run a butter knife around the edges before removing to make sure the crust is not stuck to the loaf pan. Cut into rectangles.

Leftover Tip: If you have leftover marmalade, use it to sweeten yogurt or oatmeal or as a topping for pancakes. If you don't have any berries on hand or don't have time to make homemade marmalade, you can use your favorite store-bought jelly, marmalade, or preserve as a filling for this crumble bar.

Per Serving (1 bar): Calories: 513; Carbohydrates: 67g; Fat: 26g; Saturated Fat: 11g; Sugars: 39g; Cholesterol: 1mg; Protein: 10g; Fiber: 11g; Sodium: 538mg

Gooey Peanut Butter Chocolate Cookies

MAKES 12 COOKIES | PREP TIME: 15 MINUTES
COOK TIME: 15 MINUTES

30 MINUTES OR LESS • DAIRY-FREE • VEGAN • VEGETARIAN

Made with whole-food ingredients and sweetened just enough to satisfy your taste buds while maintaining balanced blood sugar, these cookies are good for both your health and your happiness. They contain fiber-rich ingredients like peanut butter, flaxseed, and oats, which means there's no guilt if you eat more than one.

½ cup extra-virgin olive oil

¼ cup crunchy or smooth
    peanut butter

½ cup dark brown sugar

¼ cup coconut sugar, white
    sugar, or raw sugar

2 tablespoons ground flaxseed

6 tablespoons
    room-temperature water

2 teaspoons vanilla extract

1 cup old-fashioned oats (or oats of
    choice)

1 cup all-purpose flour

1 cup whole-wheat pastry flour or
    gluten-free flour

1 teaspoon baking soda

½ teaspoon baking powder

½ teaspoon salt

½ cup semi-sweet or dark
    chocolate chips

¼ cup slivered or roughly
    chopped almonds

1. Preheat the oven to 375°F. Line a baking sheet with parchment paper and set aside.
2. In a large bowl, cream together the oil, peanut butter, brown sugar, and coconut sugar until well combined and fluffy. Set aside.
3. In a small bowl, combine the flaxseed, water, and vanilla and set aside.
4. In a medium bowl, whisk together the oats, all-purpose flour, pastry flour, baking soda, baking powder, and salt.
5. Add the flax mixture to the peanut butter mixture and use a spatula to mix together until combined.

6. Add the dry ingredients to the creamed mixture and mix together until a dough is formed, making sure not to overmix. Once the dough is formed, gently fold the chocolate chips and almonds into the batter.

7. Using a tablespoon or small ice-cream scoop, portion out the cookie dough into balls. Use your hands to gently roll the dough into balls.

8. Place the cookie dough balls about 1 inch apart on the prepared baking sheet.

9. Bake for 10 to 12 minutes, depending on how brown and chewy you like your cookies.

Substitution Tip: If you don't have ground flaxseed, you can substitute 1 egg. If you are allergic to peanuts, you may substitute almond butter, cashew butter, hazelnut butter, sunflower seed butter, or tahini.

Per Serving (1 cookie): Calories: 288; Carbohydrates: 36g; Fat: 14g; Saturated Fat: 2g; Sugars: 14g; Cholesterol: 0mg; Protein: 6g; Fiber: 3g; Sodium: 207mg

Olive Oil Fig Cupcakes

MAKES 12 CUPCAKES | PREP TIME: 10 MINUTES
COOK TIME: 20 MINUTES

30 MINUTES OR LESS • NUT-FREE • VEGETARIAN

The inspiration for these cupcakes came from my daily visits to my favorite coffee shop in the East Village in New York City, where they make the most delightful olive oil cake. These cupcakes are made using whole-wheat flour and ground flaxseed, which provide fiber. Lightly sweetened, these cupcakes provide all the comfort you need to satisfy your sweet tooth.

½ cup extra-virgin olive oil, plus more for greasing

1½ cups whole-wheat flour, all-purpose flour, or gluten-free flour

½ teaspoon baking soda

½ teaspoon baking powder

¼ teaspoon salt

2 teaspoons ground flaxseed

6 tablespoons room-temperature water

¾ cup milk (dairy or plant-based)

¾ cup coconut sugar or white sugar

3 teaspoons finely grated orange zest

¼ cup dried figs, roughly chopped

1. Preheat the oven to 350°F. Line a 12-cup muffin tin with paper liners and grease the liners with oil.
2. In a medium bowl, whisk together the flour, baking soda, baking powder, and salt.
3. In a small bowl, whisk together the flaxseed, water, and milk until well incorporated and gooey.
4. In a large bowl, cream together the ½ cup of oil and the sugar until well combined. Add the orange zest.
5. Add the flaxseed mixture to the creamed oil-and-sugar mixture, and then gradually add the dry ingredients and continue to mix until incorporated, making sure not to overmix.

6. Fold the dried figs into the cupcake batter, making sure all the figs are well incorporated. Using a spoon or ice-cream scooper, spoon the batter into the muffin cups.
7. Bake for 20 minutes, or until you stick a toothpick into the cupcake and it comes out clean.

Technique Tip: To make sure the cupcakes are evenly baked, rotate the pan about halfway through baking. Poke one cupcake with a toothpick to make sure it is done. If the toothpick is wet after submerging into the cupcake, cook for 2 to 3 minutes more.

Per Serving (1 cupcake): Calories: 201; Carbohydrates: 26g; Fat: 10g; Saturated Fat: 2g; Sugars: 15g; Cholesterol: 0mg; Protein: 3g; Fiber: 2g; Sodium: 110mg

Carrot Cake Scones

MAKES 15 SCONES | PREP TIME: 15 MINUTES
COOK TIME: 20 MINUTES

NUT-FREE · VEGAN · VEGETARIAN

I adore the concept of tea and scones for dessert. When I created this dessert, I combined two of my favorite treats—scones and carrot cake. These scones are very lightly sweetened and derive most of their natural sweetness from the raisins, carrots, and Granny Smith apples used in the recipe. This recipe is perfect proof that healthy can also be scrummy.

2½ cups whole-wheat pastry flour, all-purpose flour, or gluten-free flour

2 teaspoons ground cinnamon

1½ teaspoons baking powder

1 teaspoon baking soda

1 teaspoon ground nutmeg

¼ teaspoon sea salt

½ cup milk (dairy or planted-based)

5 tablespoons maple syrup

¼ cup raisins

Zest of 1 lemon

1 tablespoon lemon juice

4 tablespoons extra-virgin olive oil

½ cup grated carrots

½ cup grated Granny Smith apple

1. Preheat the oven to 350°F. Line a baking sheet with parchment paper and set aside.
2. In a medium bowl, whisk together the flour, cinnamon, baking powder, baking soda, nutmeg, and salt.
3. In a small bowl, combine the milk, maple syrup, raisins, lemon zest, and lemon juice. Whisk and set aside.
4. Add the oil to the flour mixture, using a whisk to incorporate.
5. Pour the milk mixture into the oil-and-flour mixture, and use a spatula to gently mix until just combined, being careful to not overmix. Gently fold in the carrots and apple.
6. Using a spoon or an ice-cream scoop, drop 1-inch balls of dough onto the prepared baking sheet about 1 inch apart.

7. Bake for about 8 minutes, then rotate the baking sheet in the oven and continue to bake for 6 to 8 minutes more, or until golden on top and somewhat firm to the touch.

8. Remove the baking sheet from the oven and transfer the scones to a cooling rack. Serve warm or cool and store in a sealed container in the refrigerator for up to 5 days.

Storage Tip: Before storing scones, make sure that they are completely cooled to prevent molding. These carrot scones will keep at room temperature for a couple of days, or you can store them in the refrigerator and toast them before serving.

Per Serving (1 scone): Calories: 132; Carbohydrates: 22g; Fat: 4g; Saturated Fat: 1g; Sugars: 6g; Cholesterol: 0mg; Protein: 3g; Fiber: 3g; Sodium: 131mg

Beetroot Chickpea Hummus

KES 2 CUPS | PREP TIME: 10 MINUTES

INUTES OR LESS · **DAIRY-FREE** · **GLUTEN-FREE** · **NUT-FREE** · **.N** · **VEGETARIAN**

This stunningly beautiful hummus is the perfect dip to keep in your refrigerator at all times. It's an excellent protein- and fiber-rich snack or side dish. You can also use hummus as a creamy spread for sandwiches or mix it into a salad as a dressing. Chickpeas have a low glycemic index, meaning that they do not cause a spike in blood sugar levels. Beets are rich in nitrates, which may help lower blood pressure and risk for heart disease.

1 (15-ounce) can chickpeas, drained and rinsed (save the chickpea liquid)

1 cup cooked beetroot, canned or freshly cooked

1 garlic clove

2 tablespoons aquafaba (reserved canned chickpea water), plus more as needed

2 teaspoons extra-virgin olive oil

1 tablespoon tahini

1 tablespoon lime juice

½ teaspoon salt

In a food processor or blender, blend the chickpeas, beetroot, garlic, aquafaba, oil, tahini, lime juice, and salt until the desired consistency is reached. If needed, add more aquafaba to thin out the hummus.

Variation Tip: If you love beets, you can add more of them to your hummus. You can also experiment with adding fresh ginger to spice up your hummus; about 1 tablespoon of grated ginger works well. Also, you can swap out the lime juice for lemon if that's what you have on hand.

Per Serving (½ cup): Calories: 137; Carbohydrates: 18g; Fat: 6g; Saturated Fat: 1g; Sugars: 6g; Cholesterol: 0mg; Protein: 5g; Fiber: 5g; Sodium: 441mg

Raw Chocolate Truffles

MAKES 12 TRUFFLES | PREP TIME: 15 MINUTES

30 MINUTES OR LESS · DAIRY-FREE · GLUTEN-FREE · VEGAN · VEGETARIAN

These gooey, chewy, deliciously rich truffles are made with naturally occurring sugar found in raisins. Raisins are a good source of fiber, which is crucial for promoting healthy blood sugar levels. If you are allergic to cashews, substitute your favorite raw seeds or nuts. For an extra-chocolaty flavor, add an extra 1 to 2 tablespoons of cocoa or cacao powder.

2 cups raisins

2 tablespoons water

1 cup raw cashews

1 tablespoon cocoa powder

1 teaspoon ground cinnamon

½ teaspoon vanilla extract

½ cup pumpkin seeds

¼ teaspoon salt

1. Combine the raisins and water in a food processor and pulse until a paste is formed.
2. Add the cashews, cocoa, cinnamon, and vanilla to the food processor and pulse until a paste is formed.
3. Add the pumpkin seeds and salt to the mixture and pulse until the pumpkin seeds are chopped. (Do not overprocess. You don't want the pumpkin seeds to turn into a paste.)
4. Use a spoon to scoop about 2 teaspoons of mixture and form small balls using your hands. Place on parchment paper, spaced 1 inch apart.
5. Store in an airtight container in the refrigerator or at room temperature.

Substitution Tip: You can add different spices to change up the flavor. A quarter teaspoon of powdered ginger, cardamom, and nutmeg all work great! Optionally, you can roll the truffle balls in ½ cup of cocoa powder, powdered sugar, or sesame seeds for added taste.

Per Serving (1 truffle): Calories: 172; Carbohydrates: 24g; Fat: 8g; Saturated Fat: 1g; Sugars: 15g; Cholesterol: 1mg; Protein: 10g; Fiber: 11g; Sodium: 538mg

Chocolate Cherry Malt

SERVES 4 | PREP TIME: 10 MINUTES

30 MINUTES OR LESS · GLUTEN-FREE · ONE POT · VEGETARIAN

Who can forget the childhood thrill of going to an ice-cream shop on the weekend to get your favorite malt or shake? Desserts, when eaten mindfully, can be part of a health-supportive diet. This milkshake tastes decadent yet is made with whole-food ingredients and is rich in fiber and antioxidants. Who says you can't have the best of both worlds?

2 bananas, peeled or frozen (frozen make a creamier malt)

1½ cups frozen sweetened cherries

1 cup milk (dairy or plant-based)

1 cup ice cubes

½ cup raw cashews

½ cup coconut milk

2 tablespoons cocoa powder or cacao powder

2 teaspoons vanilla extract

2 teaspoons ground cinnamon (optional)

In a blender, blend the bananas, cherries, dairy milk, ice cubes, cashews, coconut milk, cocoa, vanilla, and cinnamon (if using) until smooth. Serve immediately or pour into airtight jars for storage. The milkshake will remain fresh in the freezer for 3 to 4 days.

Variation Tip: If your blender has trouble processing the ingredients, add more milk. This recipe tastes great with 1 cup of coffee or one or more shots of espresso. If you are allergic to cashews, you can substitute almonds or simply omit the nuts.

Per Serving: Calories: 291; Carbohydrates: 34g; Fat: 16g; Saturated Fat: 8g; Sugars: 19g; Cholesterol: 5mg; Protein: 8g; Fiber: 4g; Sodium: 36mg

Banana Cashew Butter Vegan Ice Cream

SERVES 4 | PREP TIME: 15 MINUTES

30 MINUTES OR LESS · GLUTEN-FREE · DAIRY-FREE · VEGAN · VEGETARIAN

Making your own creamy, fluffy, nourishing ice cream is a simple and exciting process. Since this ice cream uses bananas as the main ingredient, it contains fiber, antioxidants, and minerals. Furthermore, bananas contain pectin, which may help balance blood sugar levels. As a general rule, I like to keep five to 10 ripe bananas in my freezer at all times so that they are always ready to go for ice cream or smoothies.

5 ripe bananas, frozen (see technique tip)

¾ cup full-fat coconut milk

¼ cup cashew butter

2 teaspoons maple syrup (optional)

2 teaspoons vanilla extract

½ teaspoon ground cinnamon (optional)

½ cup dark chocolate chips or semi-sweet chocolate chips (optional)

1. In a food processor, pulse the bananas, coconut milk, cashew butter, maple syrup, vanilla, and cinnamon (if using). Process until smooth and creamy. Add the chocolate chips (if using) to the food processor and pulse five times.
2. Serve immediately or store in a freezer-safe container in the freezer for up to 6 months. For easy storing and serving, pour the ice-cream batter into ice-pop molds.

Substitution Tip: If you don't have cashew butter handy, you can use peanut butter, almond butter, or tahini. Feel free to get creative and add a cup of berries or a tablespoon of cocoa powder to change up the flavor.

Technique Tip: To properly freeze bananas, peel the bananas and cut them into 2-inch pieces. Place the pieces in a freezer bag, and immediately sprinkle with lemon or lime juice to prevent browning.

Per Serving: Calories: 318; Carbohydrates: 40g; Fat: 18g; Saturated Fat: 10g; Sugars: 20g; Cholesterol: 0mg; Protein: 4g; Fiber: 4g; Sodium: 54mg

Measurement Conversions

	US STANDARD	US STANDARD (OUNCES)	METRIC (APPROXIMATE)
VOLUME EQUIVALENTS (LIQUID)	2 tablespoons	1 fl. oz.	30 mL
	¼ cup	2 fl. oz.	60 mL
	½ cup	4 fl. oz.	120 mL
	1 cup	8 fl. oz.	240 mL
	1½ cups	12 fl. oz.	355 mL
	2 cups or 1 pint	16 fl. oz.	475 mL
	4 cups or 1 quart	32 fl. oz.	1 L
	1 gallon	128 fl. oz.	4 L
VOLUME EQUIVALENTS (DRY)	⅛ teaspoon	————	0.5 mL
	¼ teaspoon	————	1 mL
	½ teaspoon	————	2 mL
	¾ teaspoon	————	4 mL
	1 teaspoon	————	5 mL
	1 tablespoon	————	15 mL
	¼ cup	————	59 mL
	⅓ cup	————	79 mL
	½ cup	————	118 mL
	⅔ cup	————	156 mL
	¾ cup	————	177 mL
	1 cup	————	235 mL
	2 cups or 1 pint	————	475 mL
	3 cups	————	700 mL
	4 cups or 1 quart	————	1 L
	½ gallon	————	2 L
	1 gallon	————	4 L
WEIGHT EQUIVALENTS	½ ounce	————	15 g
	1 ounce	————	30 g
	2 ounces	————	60 g
	4 ounces	————	115 g
	8 ounces	————	225 g
	12 ounces	————	340 g
	16 ounces or 1 pound	————	455 g

	FAHRENHEIT (F)	CELSIUS (C) (APPROXIMATE)
OVEN TEMPERATURES	250°F	120°C
	300°F	150°C
	325°F	180°C
	375°F	190°C
	400°F	200°C
	425°F	220°C
	450°F	230°C

Resources

CDC.gov/diabetes: Centers for Disease Control and Prevention, a government website with diabetes-specific health information

Diabetes.org: American Diabetes Association, a leading diabetes research organization

Health.Harvard.edu: Harvard Medical School, offering numerous articles with health tips and information

Heart.org: American Heart Association, offering a website with diabetes-specific information and health tips

MedlinePlus.gov/prediabetes.html: a government website with diabetes-specific health information

References

American Academy of Dermatology Association. "Diabetes: 12 Warning Signs That Appear on Your Skin." Accessed December 28, 2020. AAD .org/public/diseases/a-z/diabetes-warning-signs.

American Diabetes Association. "Learn the Genetics of Diabetes." Accessed December 28, 2020. Diabetes.org/diabetes/genetics-diabetes.

American Diabetes Association. "Smoking and Diabetes: American Diabetes Association." *Diabetes Care* 23, no. 1 (2000): 93–94. doi.org/10.2337/diacare.23.1.93.

American Diabetes Association. "Understanding A1C: Diagnosis." Accessed January 25, 2021. Diabetes.org/a1c/diagnosis.

Centers for Disease Control and Prevention. "Diabetes and Men." Last modified April 1, 2019. CDC.gov/diabetes/library/features /diabetes-and-men.html.

Centers for Disease Control and Prevention. "National Diabetes Statistics Report, 2020." Last modified August 28, 2020. CDC.gov /diabetes/data/statistics-report/index.html.

Colberg, Sheri R., Ronald J. Sigal, Bo Fernhall, Judith G. Regensteiner, Bryan J. Blissmer, Richard R. Rubin, Lisa Chasan-Taber, Ann L. Albright, and Barry Braun. "Exercise and Type 2 Diabetes: The American College of Sports Medicine and the American Diabetes Association: Joint Position Statement." *Diabetes Care* 33, no. 12 (2010): e147–67. doi: 10.2337/dc10-9990.

Endocrine Society. "Raising Low Vitamin D Levels Lowers Risk of Prediabetes Progressing to Diabetes." Published June 21, 2014. Endocrine.org/news-and-advocacy/news-room/2014/raising-low -vitamin-d-levels-lowers-risk-of-prediabetes-progressing-to-diabetes.

Francois, Monique E., and Jonathan P. Little. "Effectiveness and Safety of High-Intensity Interval Training in Patients with Type 2 Diabetes." *Diabetes Spectrum* no. 1 (January 2015): 39–44. NCBI.NLM.NIH.gov /pmc/articles/PMC4334091.

Freemantle, N., J. Holmes, A. Hockey, and S. Kumar. "How Strong Is the Association between Abdominal Obesity and the Incidence of

Type 2 Diabetes?" *International Journal of Clinical Practice* 62, no. 9 (2008): 1391–96. doi: 10.1111/j.1742-1241.2008.01805.x.

Grandner, Michael A., Azizi Seixas, Safal Shetty, and Sundeep Shenoy. "Sleep Duration and Diabetes Risk: Population Trends and Potential Mechanisms." *Current Diabetes Reports* 16, no. 11 (2016): 106. NCBI.NLM.NIH.gov/pmc/articles/PMC5070477.

Harvard Health Publishing. "Exercising to Relax." Harvard Medical School. Last modified July 7, 2020. Health.Harvard.edu/staying -healthy/exercising-to-relax.

Hostalek, Ulrike. "Global Epidemiology of Prediabetes—Present and Future Perspectives." *Clinical Diabetes and Endocrinology* 5, no. 1 (2019): 1–5. doi: 10.1186/s40842-019-0080-0.

Hsia, Daniel S., Sandra Larrivee, William T. Cefalu, and William D. Johnson. "Impact of Lowering BMI Cut Points as Recommended in the Revised American Diabetes Association's *Standards of Medical Care in Diabetes—2015* on Diabetes Screening in Asian Americans." *Diabetes Care* 38, no. 11 (2015): 2166–68. doi: 10.2337/dc15-0299.

Huffman, Jeff C., Christina M. DuBois, Rachel A. Millstein, Christopher M. Celano, and Deborah Wexler. "Positive Psychological Interventions for Patients with Type 2 Diabetes: Rationale, Theoretical Model, and Intervention Development." *Journal of Diabetes Research* 2015, no. 3 (2015): 1–18. doi: 10.1155/2015/428349.

Jung, Suk Hwa, Kyoung Hwa Ha, and Dae Jung Kim. "Visceral Fat Mass Has Stronger Associations with Diabetes and Prediabetes Than Other Anthropometric Obesity Indicators among Korean Adults." *Yonsei Medical Journal* 57, no. 3 (2016): 674–80. doi.org/10.3349 /ymj.2016.57.3.674.

Kautzky-Willer, Alexandra, Jürgen Harreiter, and Giovanni Pacini. "Sex and Gender Differences in Risk, Pathophysiology and Complications of Type 2 Diabetes Mellitus." *Endocrine Reviews* 37, no. 3 (June 2016): 278–316. doi: 10.1210/er.2015-1137.

Kim, Kyoung-Yun, and Jeong Seop Park. "Impact of Fish Consumption by Subjects with Prediabetes on the Metabolic Risk Factors: Using Data in the 2015 (6th) Korea National Health and Nutrition Examination Surveys." *Nutrition Research and Practice* 12, no. 3 (2018): 233–42. doi: 10.4162/nrp.2018.12.3.233.

Kirkman, M. Sue, Vanessa Jones Briscoe, Nathaniel Clark, Hermes Florez, Linda B. Haas, Jeffrey B. Halter, Elbert S. Huang et al. "Diabetes in Older Adults: Consensus Report." *Journal of the American Geriatrics Society* 60, no. 12 (2012): 2342–56. doi: 10.1111/jgs.12035.

MedlinePlus. "Diabetes Complications." National Institutes of Health. Last modified December 10, 2020. MedlinePlus.gov/diabetes complications.html.

National Institute of Diabetes and Digestive and Kidney Diseases. "Recommended Tests for Identifying Prediabetes." Accessed January 25, 2021. NIDDK.NIH.gov/health-information/professionals /clinical-tools-patient-management/diabetes/game-plan-preventing -type-2-diabetes/prediabetes-screening-how-why/recommended -tests-identifying-prediabetes.

National Institutes of Health. "Physical Activity May Reduce Depression Symptoms." Published January 15, 2019. NIH.gov/news-events/nih -research-matters/physical-activity-helps-reduce-depression -symptoms.

Pacheco, Danielle. "Lack of Sleep and Diabetes." Sleep Foundation. Last modified November 10, 2020. SleepFoundation.org/physical -health/lack-of-sleep-and-diabetes.

Reynolds, Andrew N., Ashley P. Akerman, and Jim Mann. "Dietary Fibre and Whole Grains in Diabetes Management: Systematic Review and Meta-Analyses." *PLoS Medicine* 17, no. 3 (2020): e1003053. doi: 10.1371/journal.pmed.1003053.

Shan, Zhilei, Hongfei Ma, Manling Xie, Peipei Yan, Yanjun Guo, Wei Bao, Ying Rong, Chandra L. Jackson, Frank B. Hu, and Liegang Liu. "Sleep Duration and Risk of Type 2 Diabetes: A Meta-analysis of Prospective Studies." *Diabetes Care* 38, no. 3 (March 2015): 529–37. doi: 10.2337 /dc14-2073.

U.S. Food and Drug Administration. "Cigarette Smoking: A Risk Factor for Type 2 Diabetes." Last modified May 4, 2020. FDA.gov/tobacco -products/health-information/cigarette-smoking-risk-factor-type-2 -diabetes.

World Health Organization. "Physical Activity." Published November 26, 2020. WHO.int/news-room/fact-sheets/detail/physical-activity.

Index

Acknowledgments

I would like to express my gratitude to my mom, Maria Teresa, my brother, Isaac, and my dad, Enrique, for empowering me to pursue my professional goals. The ultimate feminists, my family always believed in my ability to excel at anything I set my mind and heart to. Their unwavering support fuels my passion for food and nutrition advocacy. I'd also like to thank them for helping me shop for ingredients and recipe testing. This book was truly a family effort. It's important for me to acknowledge the food traditions that I inherited from my grandmothers, Abuela Alicia and Mama Chagua (Isaura). Their love for cooking using traditional Latin American ingredients has enriched my cooking philosophy. Lastly, I'd like to thank my patients for inspiring me to create recipes that are happy and healthy.

About the Author

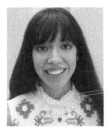 **ALICE FIGUEROA, MPH, RDN, CDN,** is a Registered Dietitian Nutritionist, National Diabetes Prevention Program Lifestyle Coach, and Public Health Research Fellow who is passionate about promoting universal access to nutrition support, health services, and wholesome foods for all segments of our global community. She is an award-winning Natural Foods Chef recognized with a James Beard Foundation National Scholars Award, as well as a Certified Yoga teacher. Her goal is to empower her patients to achieve optimum well-being through plant-based cooking, mindful nutrition, mindfulness, and intuitive and happy eating. Passionate about making nutrition accessible for all, Alice is dedicated to creating science-based nutrition content and delicious, health-supportive recipes in English, Spanish, and Portuguese, which she shares in her blog AliceInFoodieland.com. You can connect with Alice for weekly nutrition tips, public health education, and recipes through her social media accounts, including her Twitter (@alicefoodieland) and Instagram (@aliceinfoodieland) accounts.